INFOGRAPHICAL
REMEDY

Health Problems
Prevention and Remedies Institutionally & Naturally

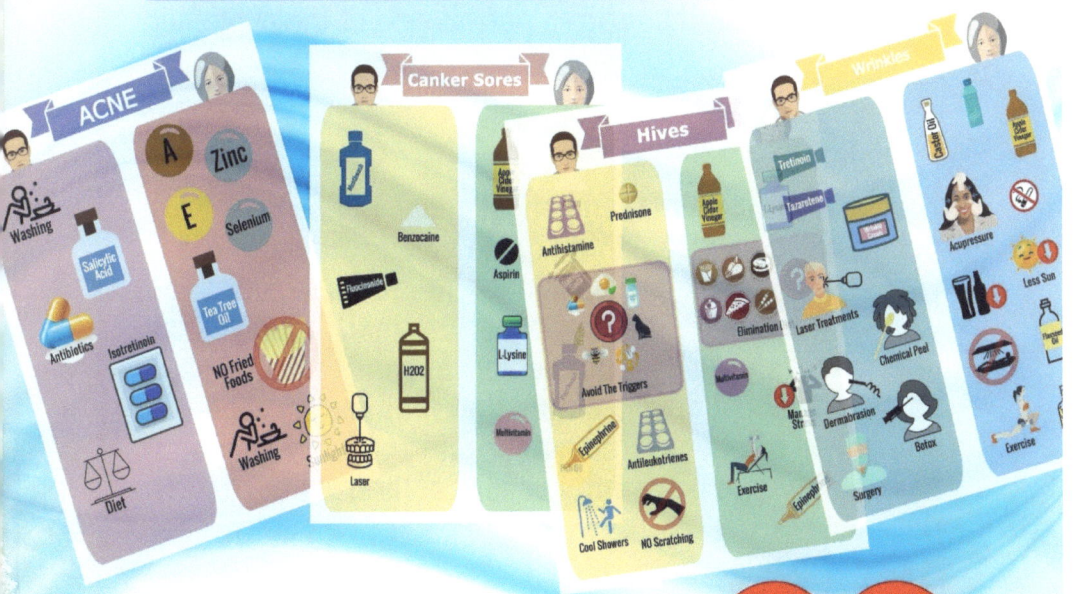

SALMAN SHARIFF

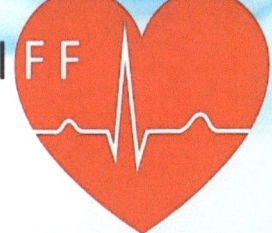

Legal Stuff

Copyright © 2017 by Salman Shariff

All rights reserved. No part of this publication may be reproduced or transmitted in any form or by any means, electronic or mechanical, including photocopying, recording, or any other information storage and retrieval system, without the written permission of the publisher.

The ideas, procedures, and suggestions in this book are not intended as a substitute for the medical advice of your trained health professional. All matters regarding your health require medical supervision. Consult your physician before adopting the suggestions in this book, as well as about any condition that may require diagnosis or medical attention. The author and publisher disclaim any liability arising directly or indirectly from the use of this book.

Medical Topics Covered

- Accidents
- Acne
- ADHD
- Age Spots
- AIDS
- Alcohol Abuse
- Allergies
- Altitude Illness
- Alzheimer's Disease
- Anal Fissures
- Anal Itching
- Anemia
- Ankle Sprain
- Anxiety
- Arthritis
- Asthma
- Athlete's Foot
- Autism
- Back Pain
- Bad Breath
- Bedsores
- Belching
- Binge Eating
- Bites & Stings
- Bladder Infections
- Blisters
- Blood Clots
- Body Odor
- Boils
- Breast Cancer
- Breast Lumps
- Bronchitis
- Bursitis
- Canker Sores
- Cataracts
- Cavities
- Cervical Dysplasia
- Chapped Lips
- Cholesterol & Triglycerides
- Cold Hands & Feet
- Colds
- Cold Sores
- Colon Cancer
- Constipation
- Calluses (Corns)
- Cough
- Dandruff
- Depression
- Dermatitis (Eczema)
- Diabetes
- Diarrhea
- Diverticulosis
- Dizziness
- Dry Hair
- Dry Eyes
- Dry Mouth
- Dry Skin
- Earache
- Erectile Dysfunction
- Fatigue
- Flatulence
- Flu
- Food Allergies
- Food Poisoning
- Foot Odor
- Foot Pain
- Gallstones
- Gastritis
- Gingivitis
- Gout
- Hair Loss
- Hangover
- Hay Fever
- Headaches
- Hearing Loss
- Heartburn
- Heart Disease
- Heart Palpitations
- Hemorrhoids
- Hepatitis
- Hiccups
- High Blood Pressure
- Hives
- Insomnia
- Irritable Bowel Syndrome
- Jock Itch
- Kidney Stones
- Knee Pain
- Laryngitis
- Low Blood Pressure
- Lung Cancer
- Lupus
- Lyme Disease
- Menopause
- Menstrual Cramps
- Mononucleosis
- Motion Sickness
- Multiple Sclerosis
- Muscle Cramps
- Nails
- Neck & Shoulder Pain
- Nightmares
- Oily Hair
- Oily Skin
- Osteoporosis
- Obesity
- Panic Attacks
- Parkinson's Disease
- Pink Eye (Conjunctivitis)
- Pneumonia
- Premature Ejaculation
- Premenstrual Syndrome
- Prostate Problems
- Psoriasis
- Rashes
- Repetitive Strain Injury
- Scars
- Sciatica
- Sinusitis
- Skin Cancer
- Sleep Apnea
- Snoring
- Sore Throat
- Stomach Pain
- Stomach Cancer
- Stress
- Stroke
- Tooth Sensitivity
- Tooth Stains
- Tumors
- Ulcers
- Urinary Tract Infections
- Varicose Veins
- Vision Problems
- Warts
- Water Retention
- Wrinkles
- Yeast Infection

IMPORTANT!

READ THIS FIRST

The goal of this book is to make you a better informed person about your health. It is a reference manual on the topic of health problems, their prevention and remedies. Use it as a guide to start your journey on treating and preventing health issues for yourself and others.

READ THIS NEXT

Do not substitute treatment by a physician with the information in this book. Use it as treatment alternatives that you can discuss with your doctor.

READ THIS ALSO

The remedies are derived from common sense and tradition going back centuries to the modern methods. They may seem ineffective initially, but are more effective and safer long-term. Not all the remedies will work on everyone. Included are remedies that have worked for people--that doesn't mean they have worked for everyone.

Using infographics is an effective technique to retain information longer than using just words alone.

The educational material presented in this book are the opinions of the author based upon years of research. Do not ignore your doctor's advice!

Companion Site

The remedies and treatments presented in this book are images so they can more easily be remembered. It is assumed that the reader can search the internet for the dosages and frequencies of the remedies. In case the reader is looking for a single source for this information, there is a website that goes along with this book.

www.infographicalremedy.com

InfograpicalRemedy.com provides more information on the remedies in this book. Please use this site to comment on your own experiences and questions you may have. The goal: a community of like-minded remedy seekers sharing and learning about conditions and their cures or remedies.

Medical topics are added periodically to the site, so check it often--or sign up on the site so you will be informed when new topics are added.

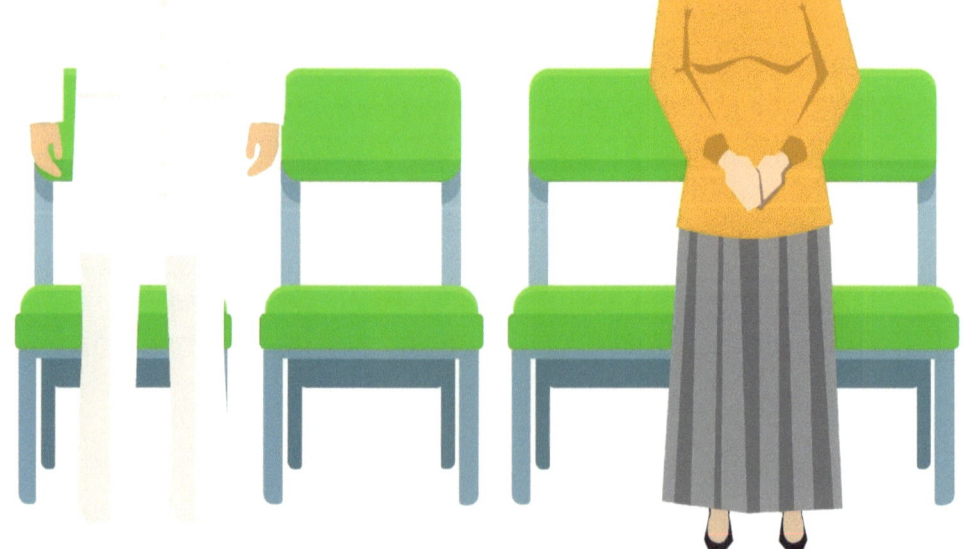

ACCIDENTS

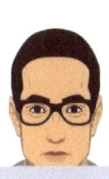
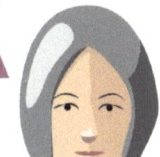
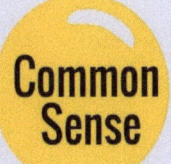
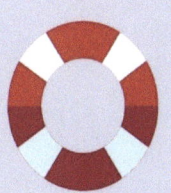
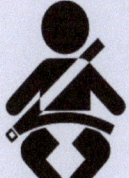
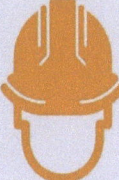

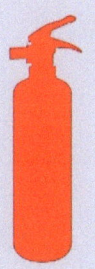
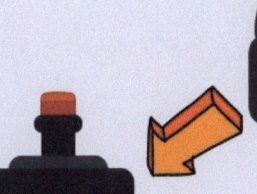
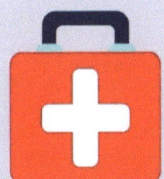

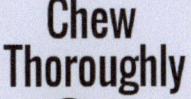

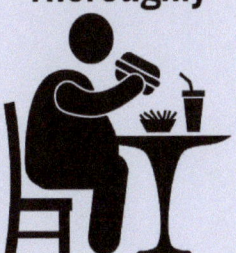

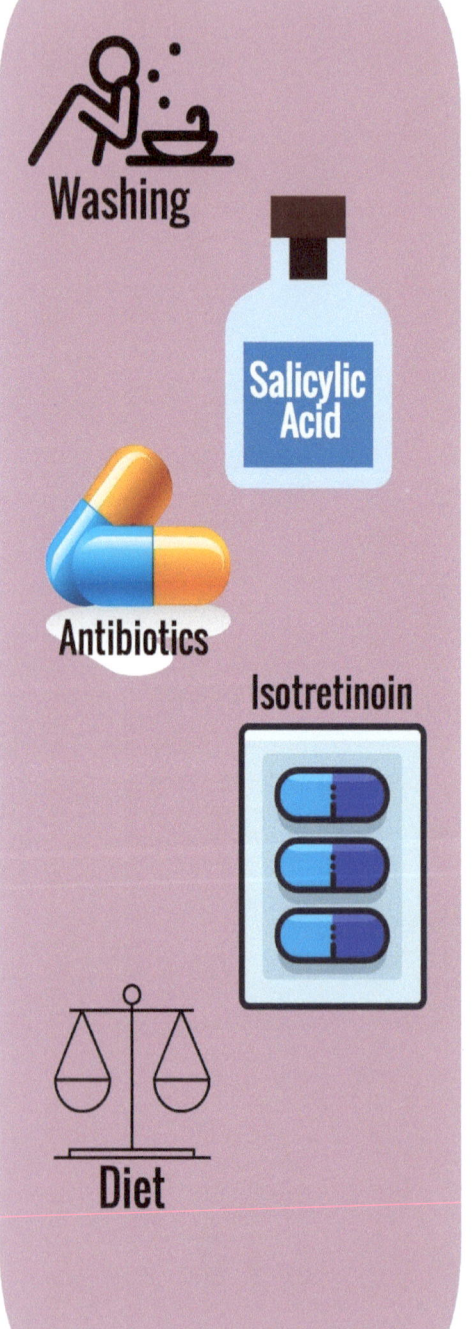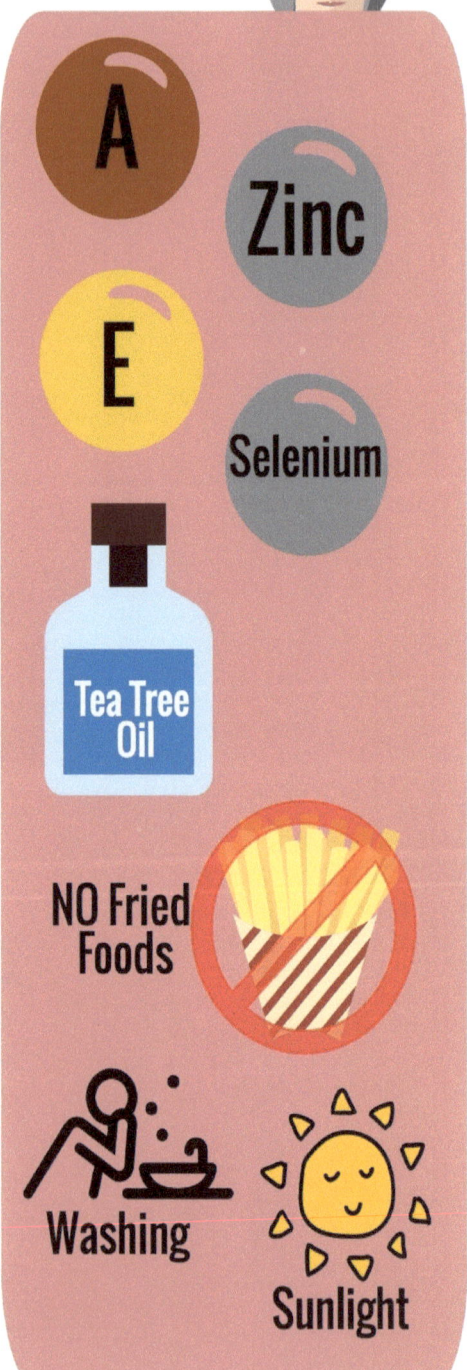

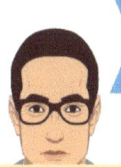 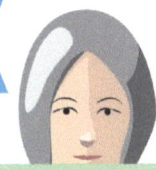

ADHD

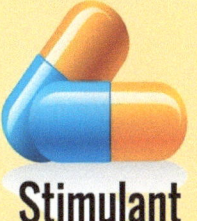
Stimulant

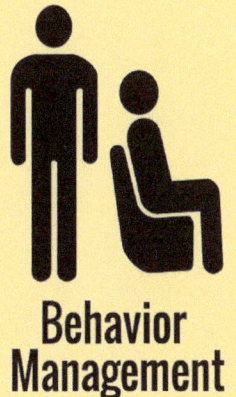
Behavior Management

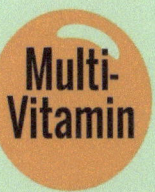
Multi-Vitamin

Fish Oil

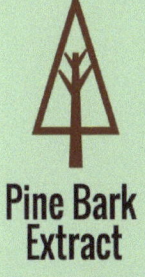
Pine Bark Extract

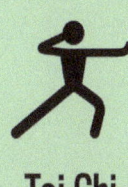
Tai Chi

NO Food Additives

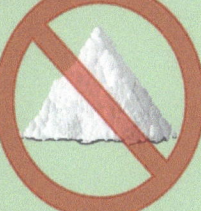
NO Sugar

NO Environmental Toxicity

Age Spots

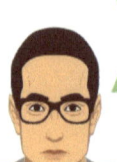
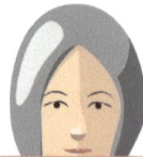

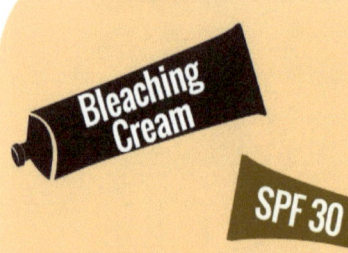

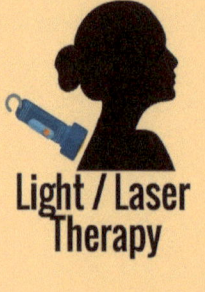
Light / Laser Therapy

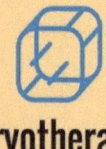
Cryotherapy

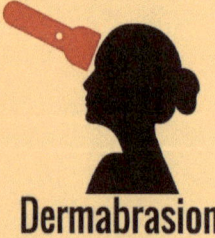
Dermabrasion

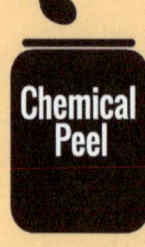
Chemical Peel

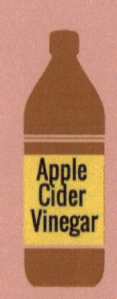
Apple Cider Vinegar

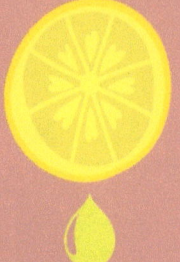
Lemon Juice

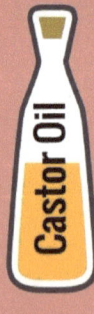
Castor Oil

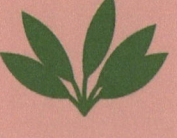
Aloe Vera

AIDS

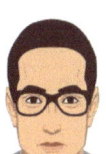
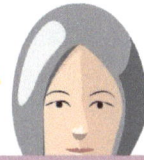

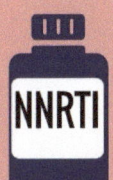 NNRTI
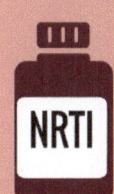 NRTI

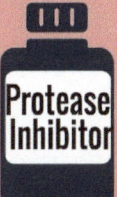 Protease Inhibitor

 Integrace Inhibitor

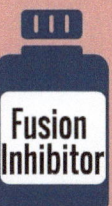 Fusion Inhibitor

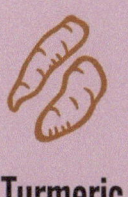
Turmeric

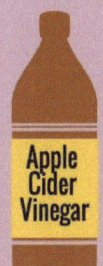 Apple Cider Vinegar

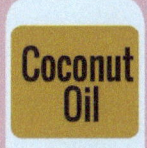 Coconut Oil

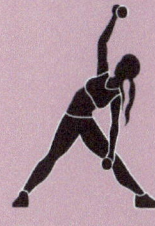

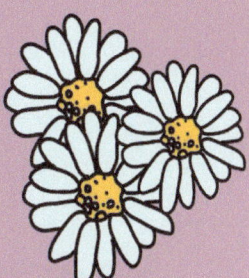
Bloodroot

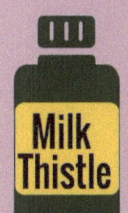 Milk Thistle

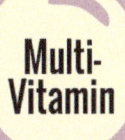 Multi-Vitamin

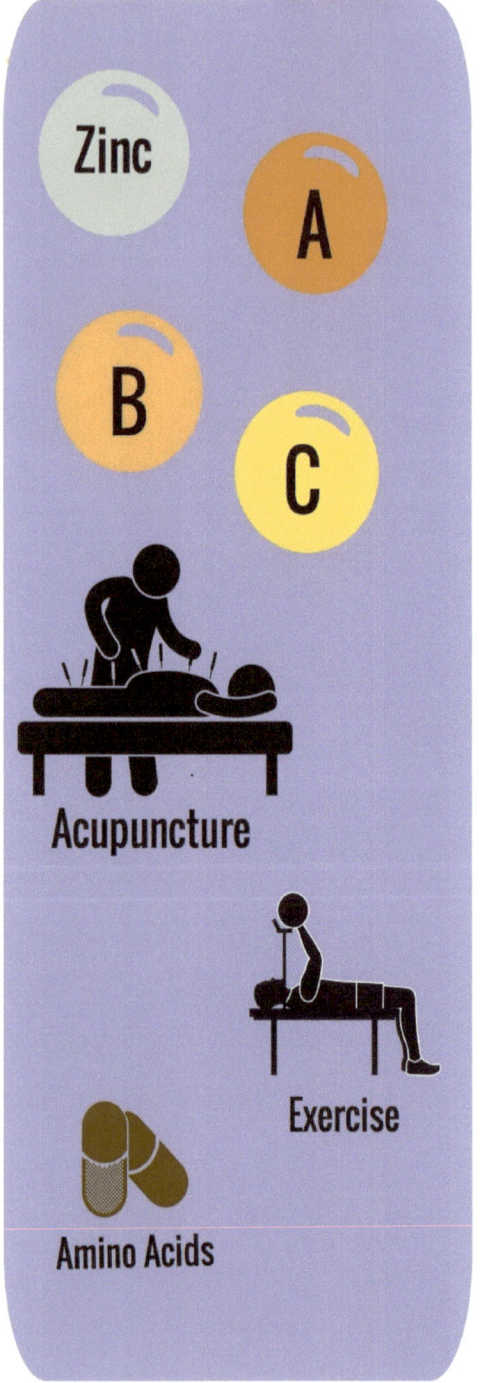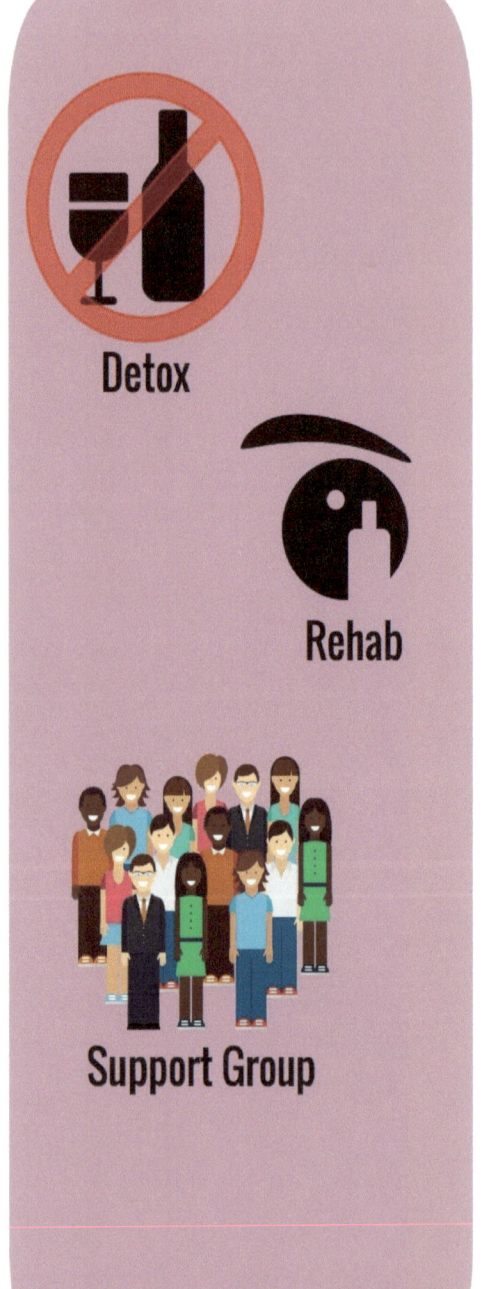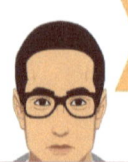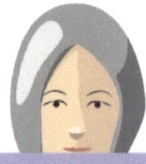

Alcoholism

- Detox
- Rehab
- Support Group
- Zinc
- A
- B
- C
- Acupuncture
- Exercise
- Amino Acids

Allergies

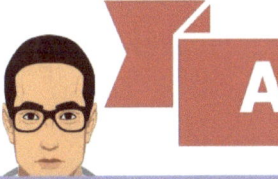
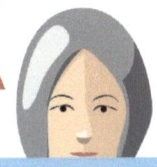

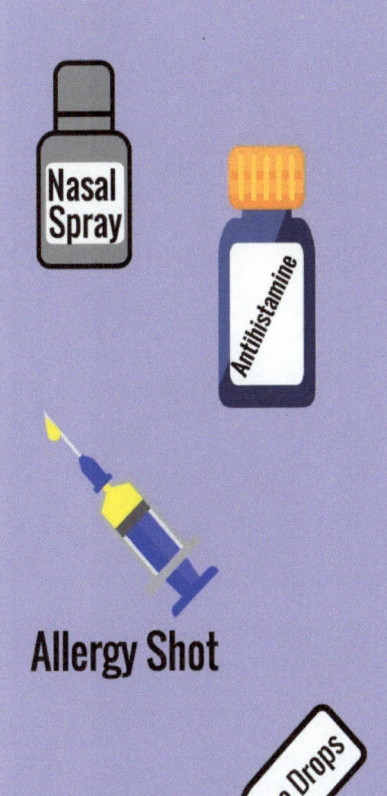

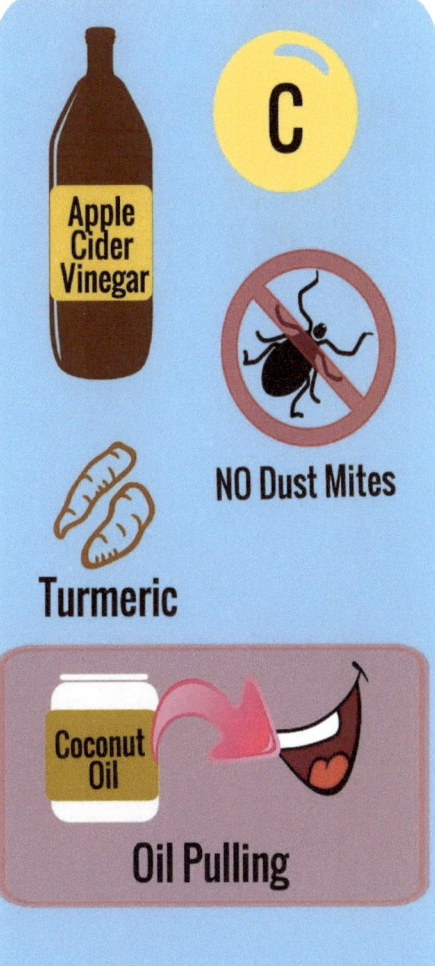

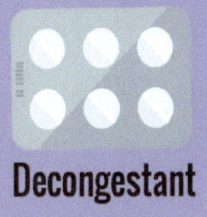

Decongestant

Honey

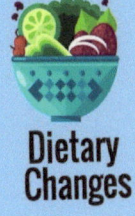
Dietary Changes

Altitude Illness

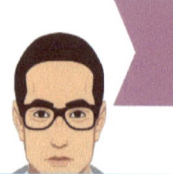
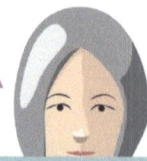
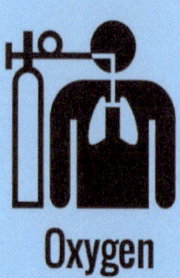

Oxygen

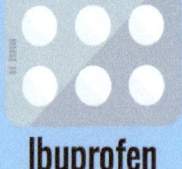

Ibuprofen

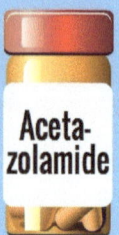

Acetazolamide

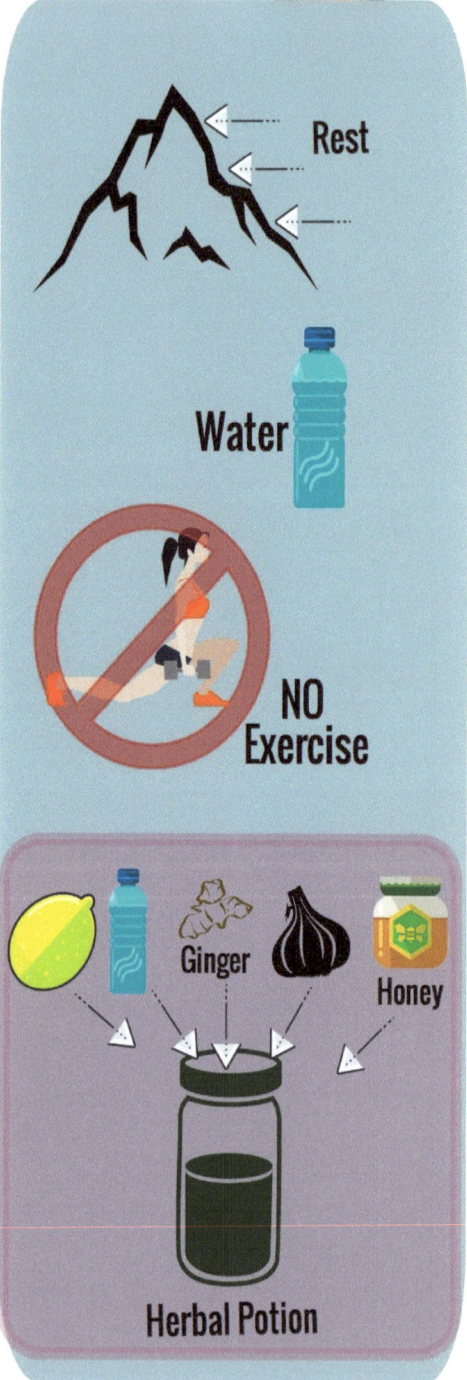

Alzheimer's Disease

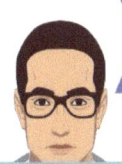
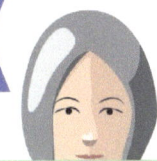

Follow Daily Routine

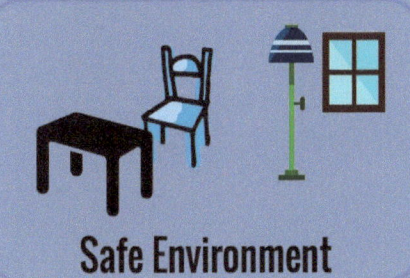
Safe Environment

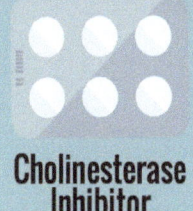
Cholinesterase Inhibitor

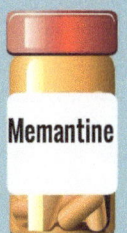
Memantine

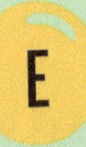 E

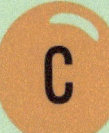 C

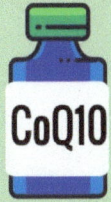 CoQ10

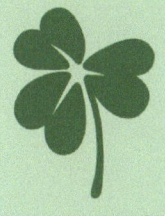 Fish Oil

Ginkgo Biloba

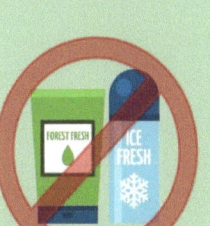
NO Aluminum

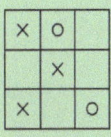
Mental Exercises

Anal Fissure

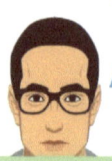
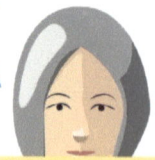

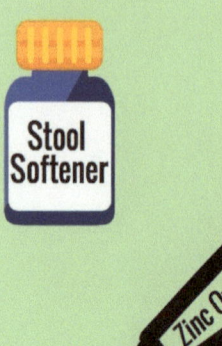
Stool Softener / Zinc Oxide

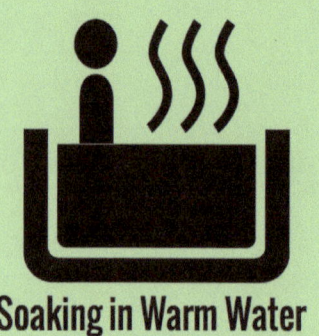
Soaking in Warm Water

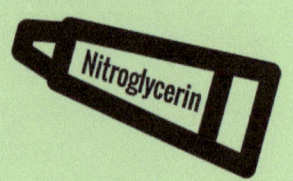
Nitroglycerin

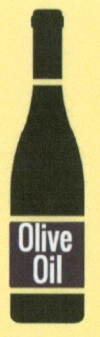
Olive Oil

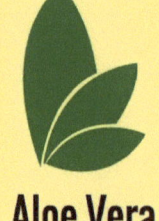
Aloe Vera

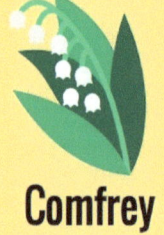
Comfrey

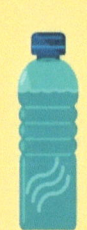

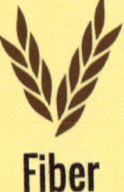
Fiber

Anal Itching

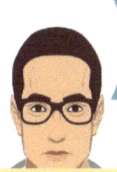
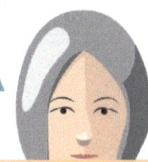

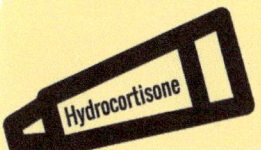

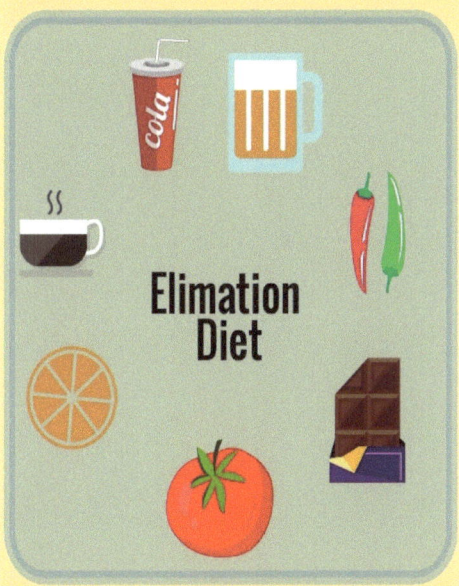
Elimation Diet

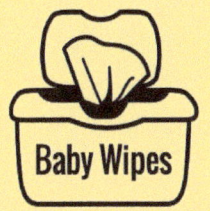
Baby Wipes

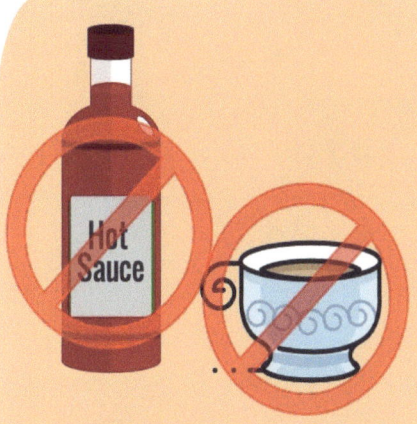
Hot Sauce

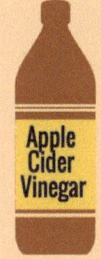
Apple Cider Vinegar

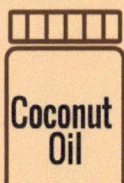
Coconut Oil

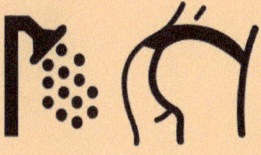

Anemia

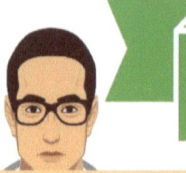
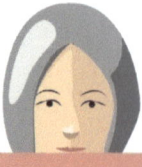

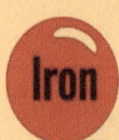 Iron
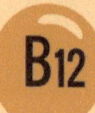 B12

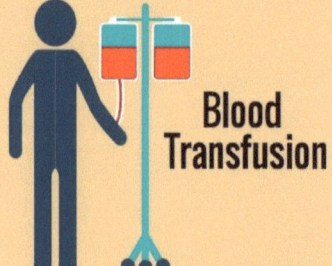 Blood Transfusion

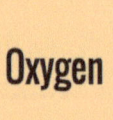 Oxygen
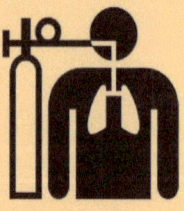

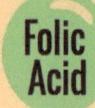 Folic Acid

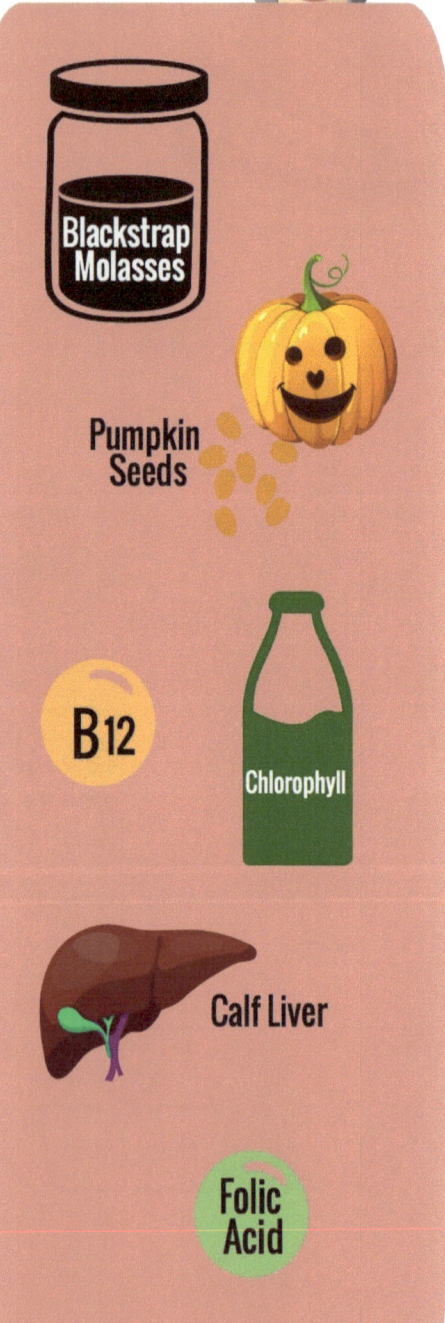

Blackstrap Molasses

Pumpkin Seeds

B12

Chlorophyll

Calf Liver

Folic Acid

Ankle Sprain

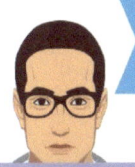
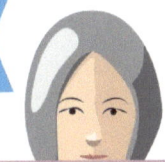
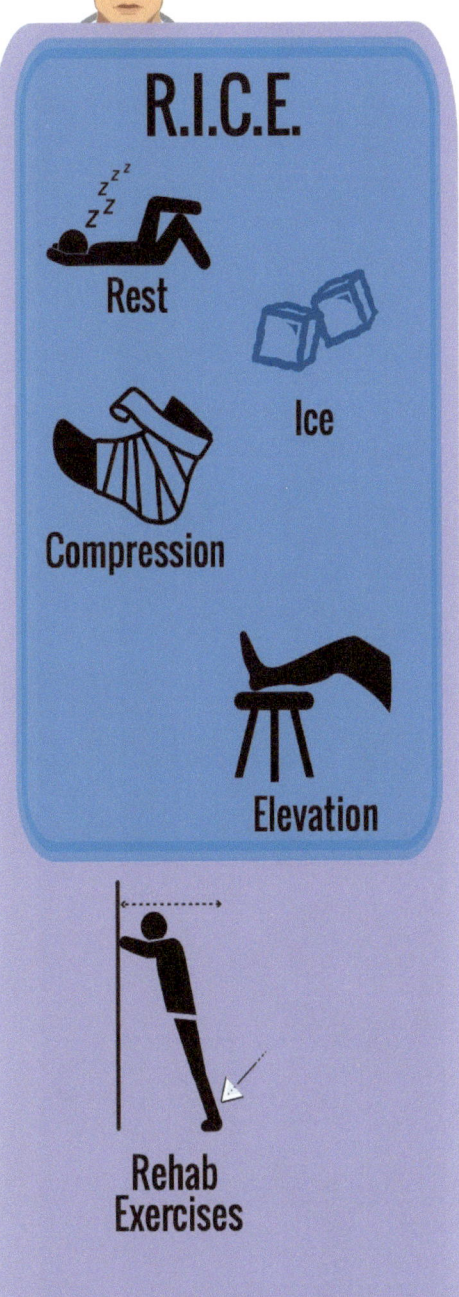
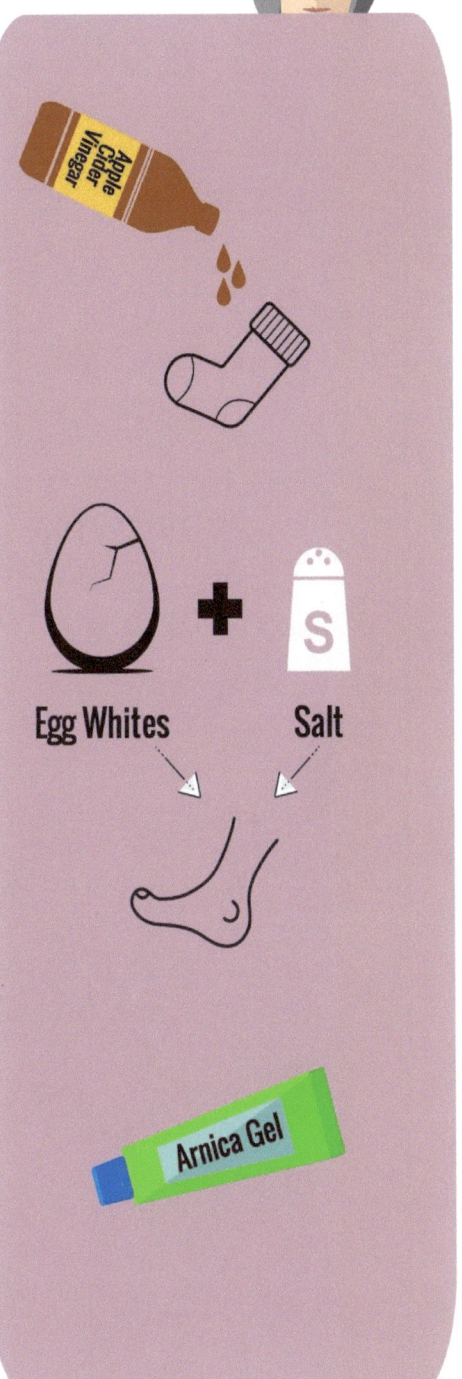

Anxiety

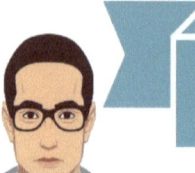
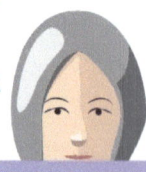
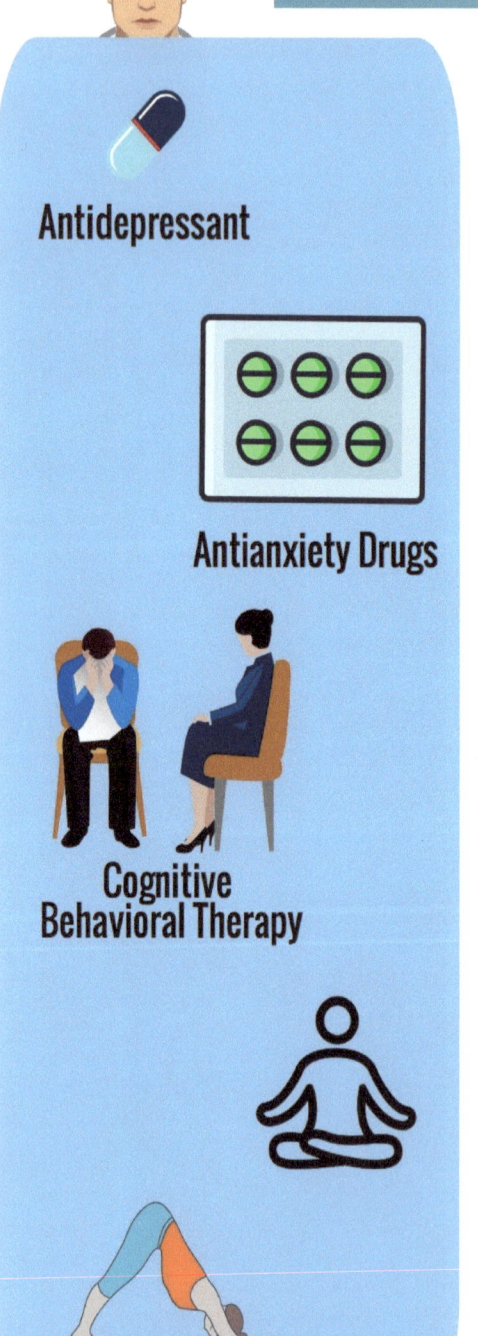
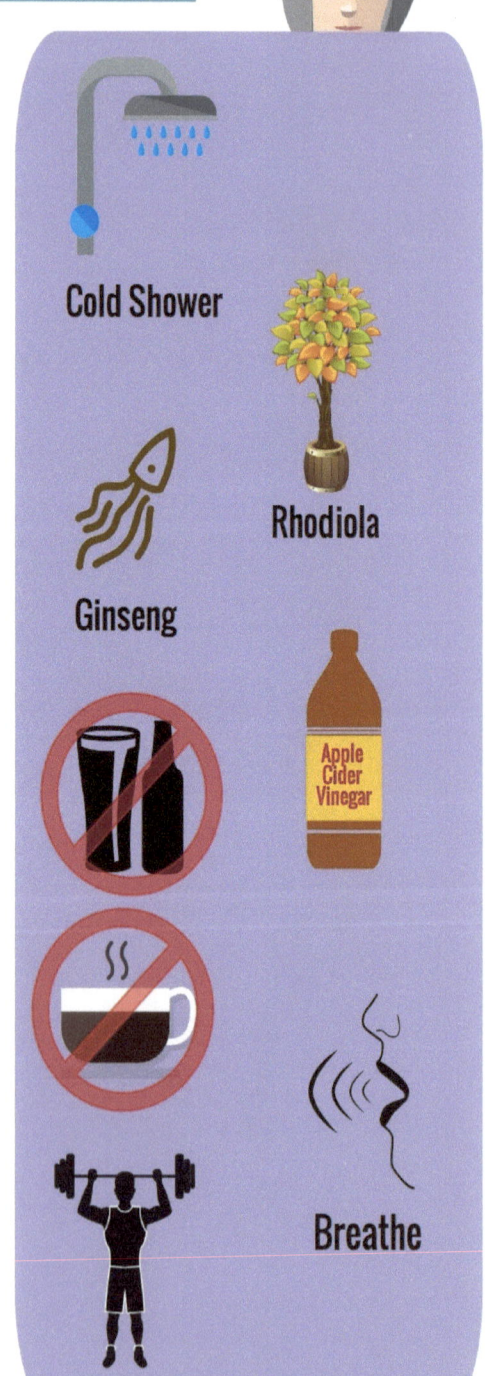

Arthritis

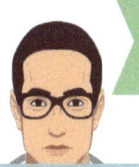
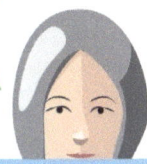
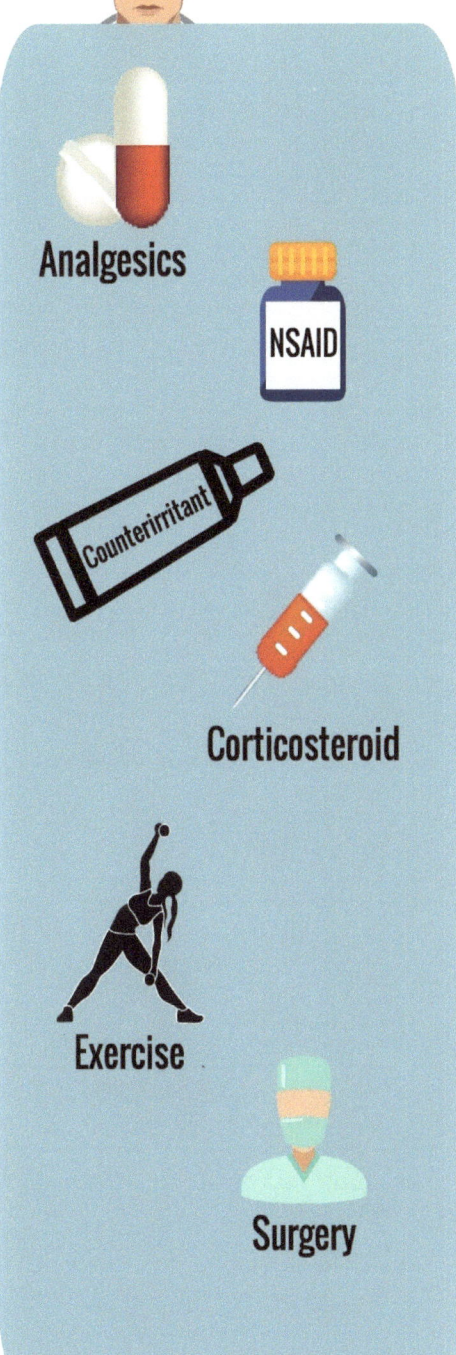
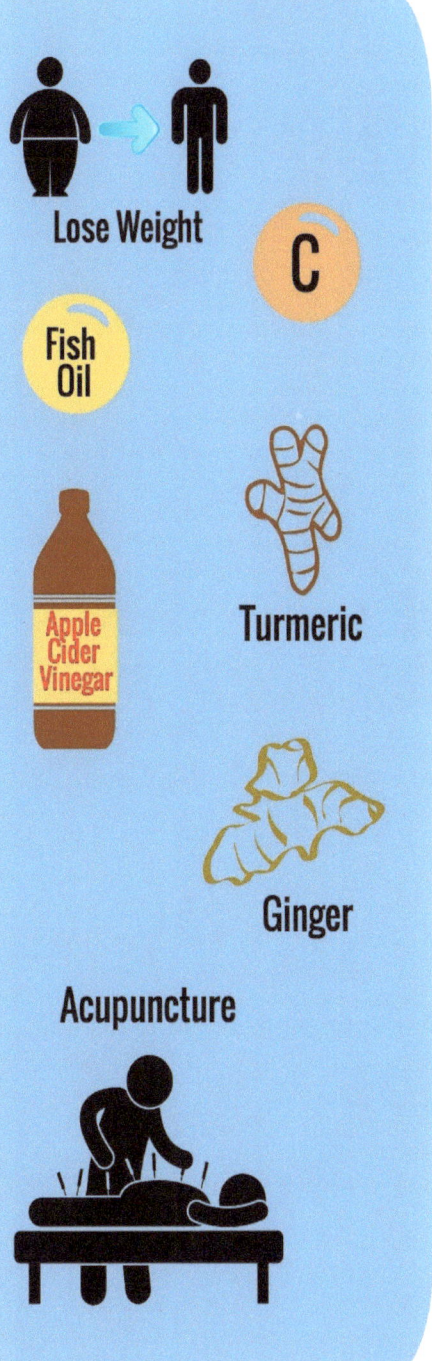

Asthma

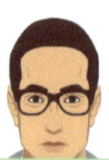
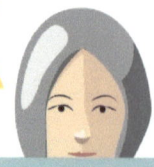
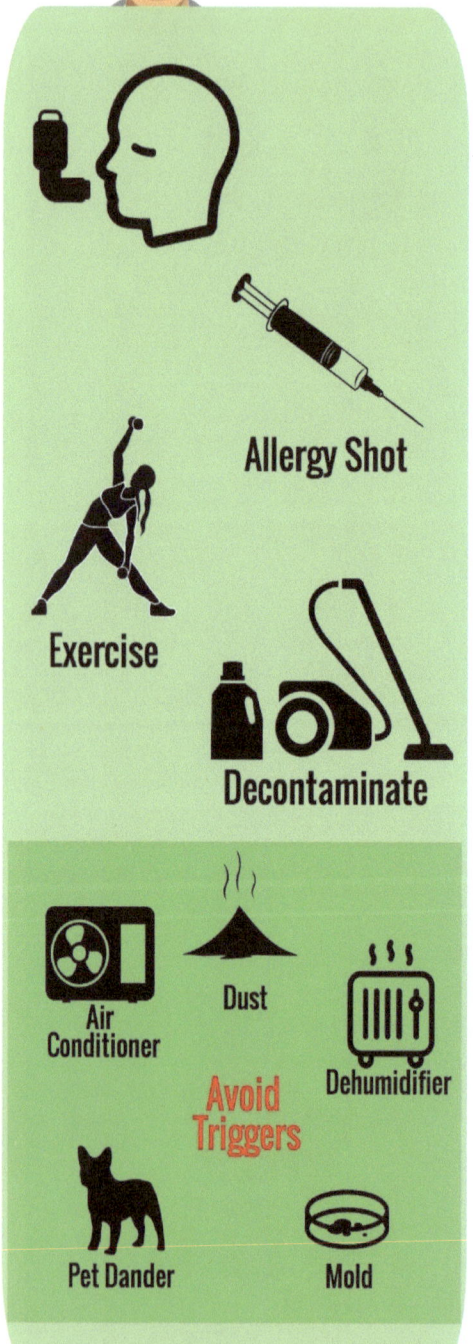
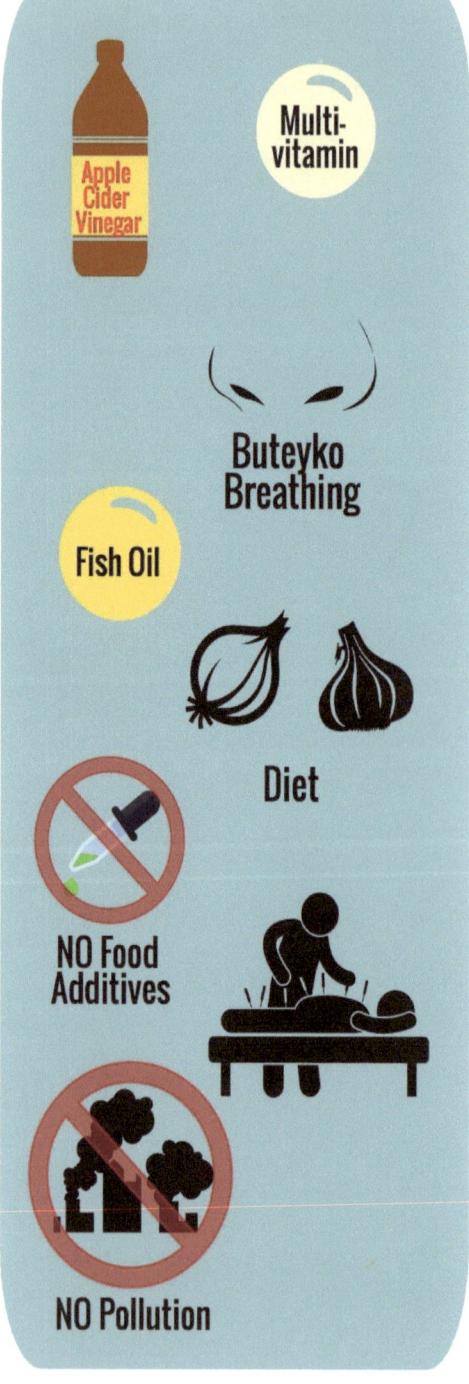

Athlete's Foot

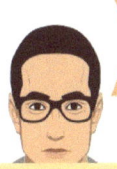
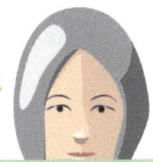

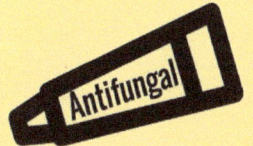

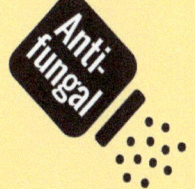

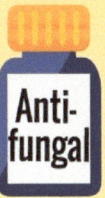

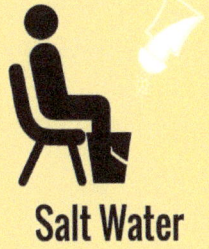

Salt Water

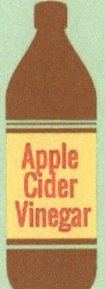

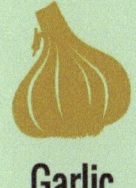

Garlic

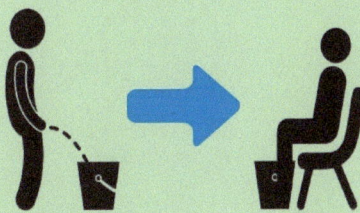

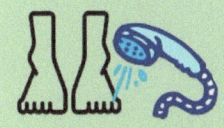

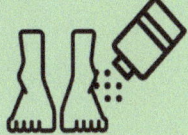

Autism

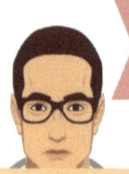
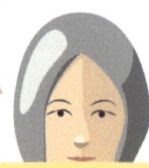

Behavior Training

Speech Therapy

SSRIs
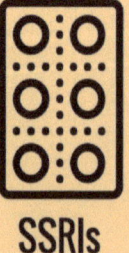

Multi-Vitamin
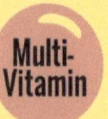

Fish Oil
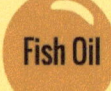

NO Gluten

NO Casein
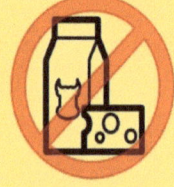

NO Food Additives

Heavy Metal Detox

Chelation Therapy
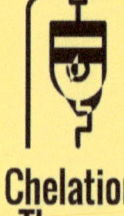

Cilantro
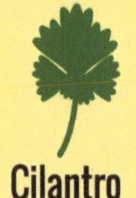

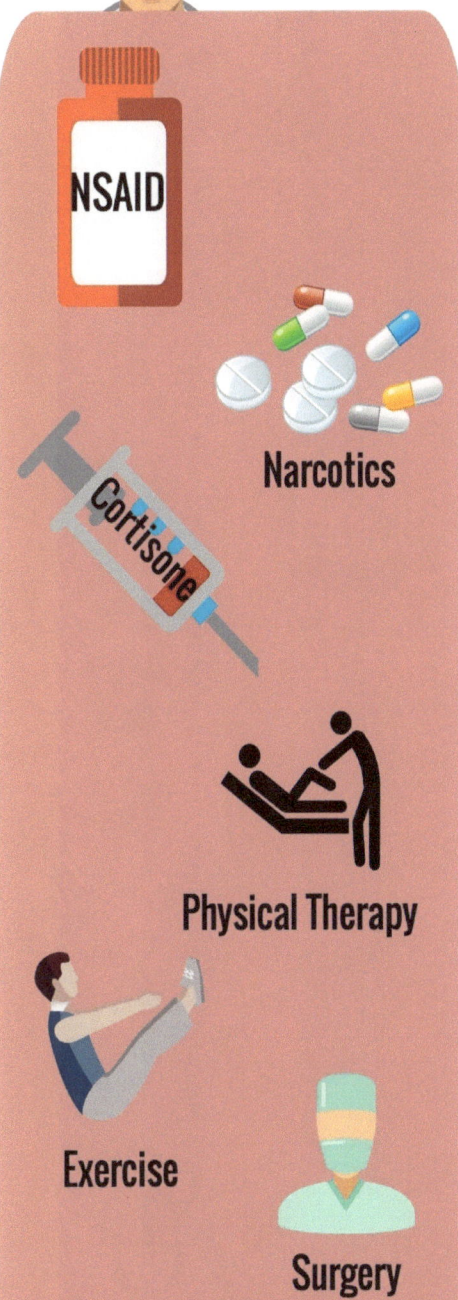

Back Pain

- NSAID
- Narcotics
- Cortisone
- Physical Therapy
- Exercise
- Surgery

- Coconut Oil
- Apple Cider Vinegar
- Stretching
- Acupuncture
- Cayenne Pepper
- Cold Shower

Bad Breath

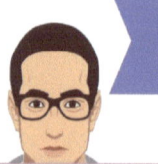
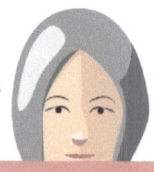
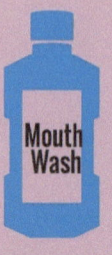
Mouth Wash

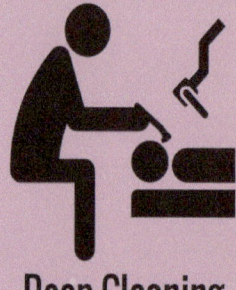
Deep Cleaning

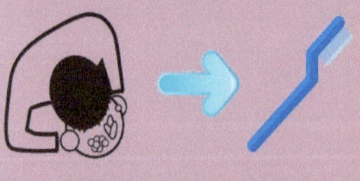
Brush After Eating

Floss

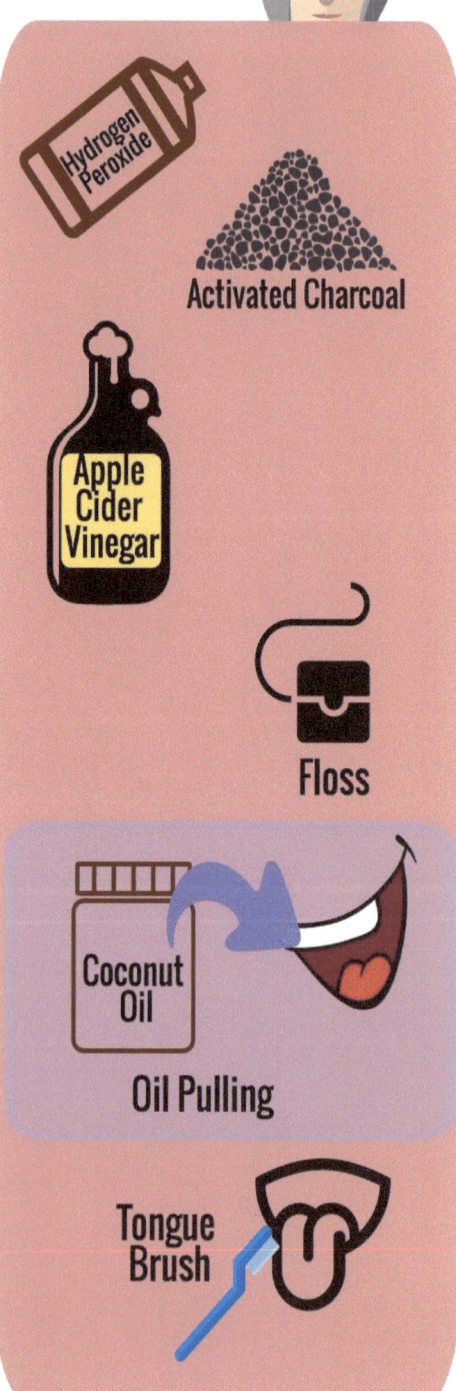
Hydrogen Peroxide

Activated Charcoal

Apple Cider Vinegar

Floss

Coconut Oil — Oil Pulling

Tongue Brush

Bedsores

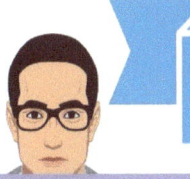
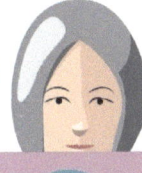

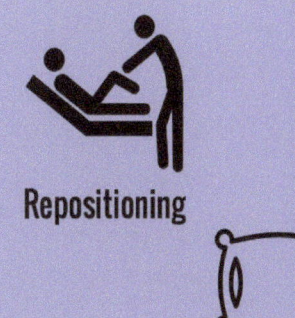
Repositioning

Relieve Pressure

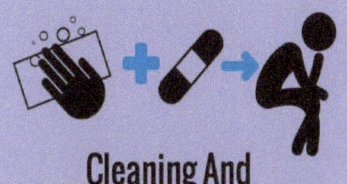
Cleaning And Dressing The Wound

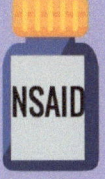
NSAID

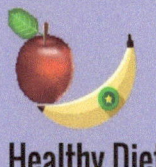
Healthy Diet

Zinc

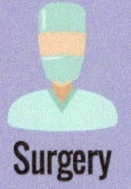
Surgery

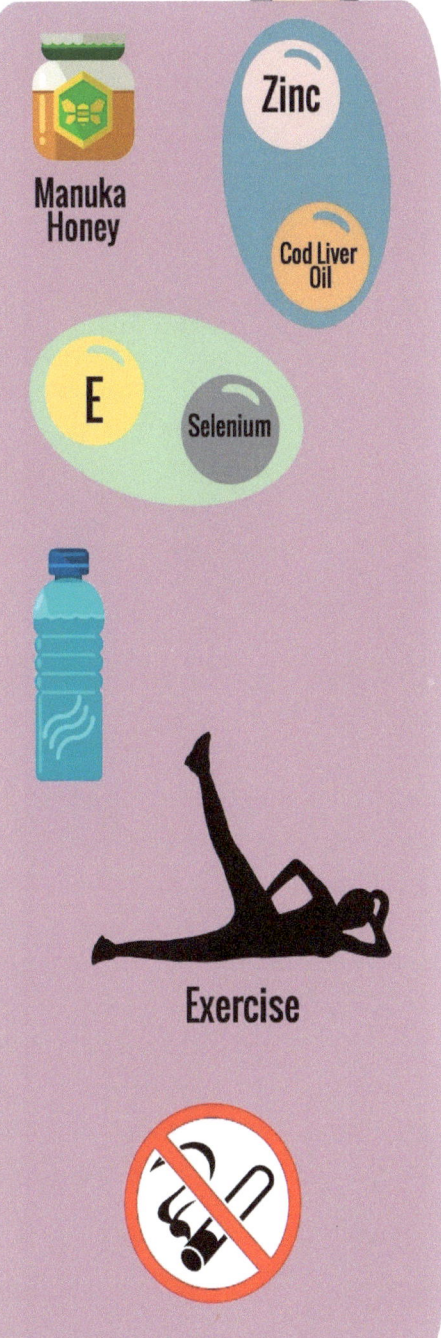

Manuka Honey

Zinc

Cod Liver Oil

E

Selenium

Exercise

Belching

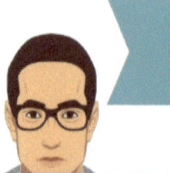
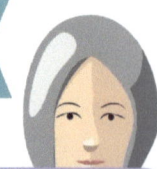
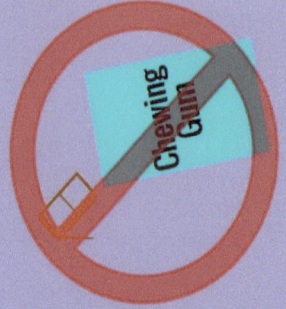
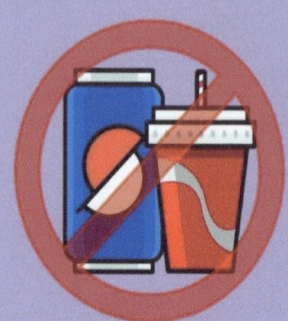

Eat Slower

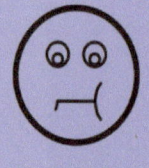
Chew More

Reduce Stress

NO Airy Foods

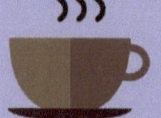 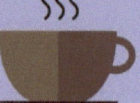
Avoid VERY Hot Beverages

Binge Eating

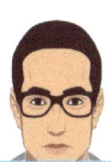
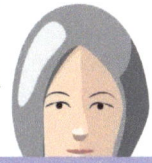

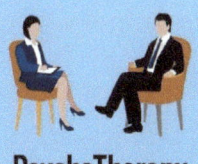
PsychoTherapy

Anti-Depressants

Appetite Suppressant

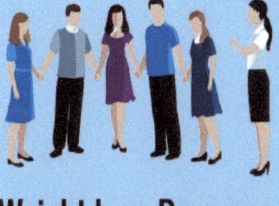
Weight Loss Programs

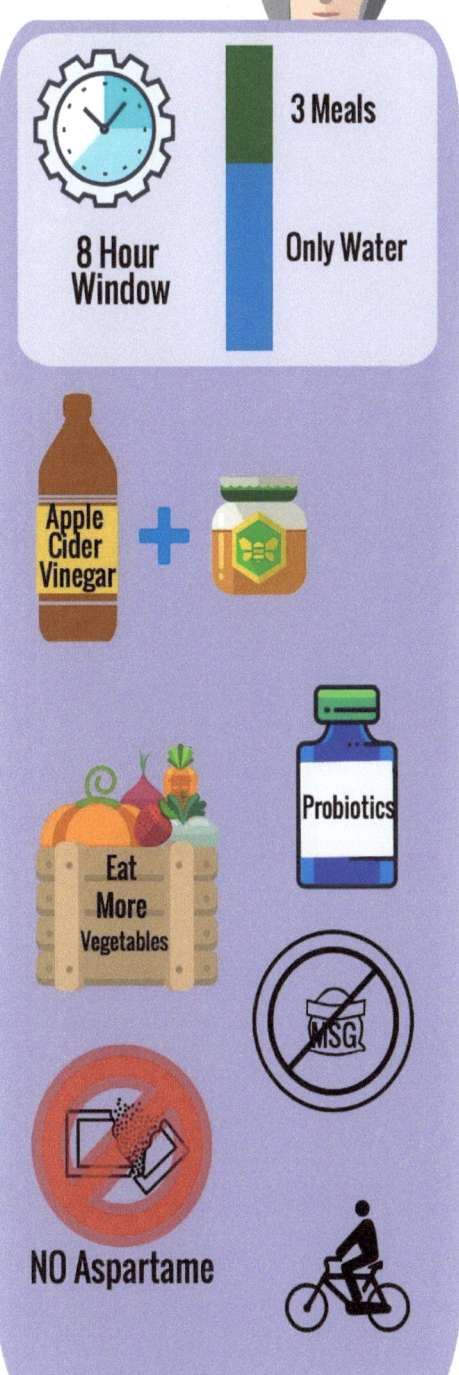

8 Hour Window | 3 Meals / Only Water

Apple Cider Vinegar +

Eat More Vegetables

Probiotics

NO Aspartame

Bites & Stings

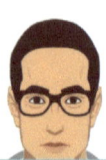
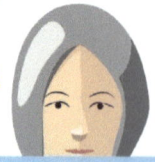
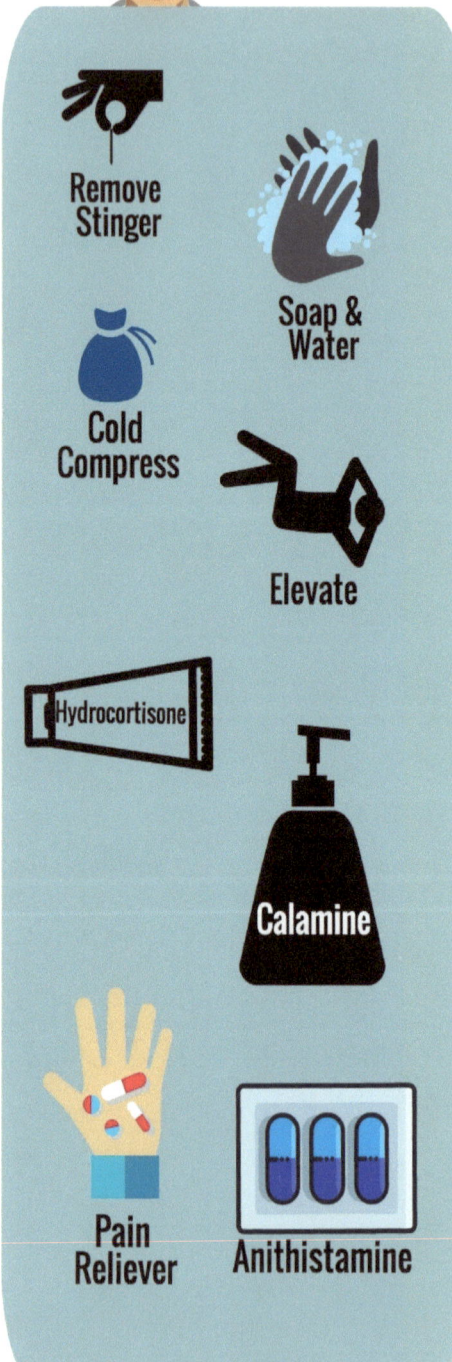
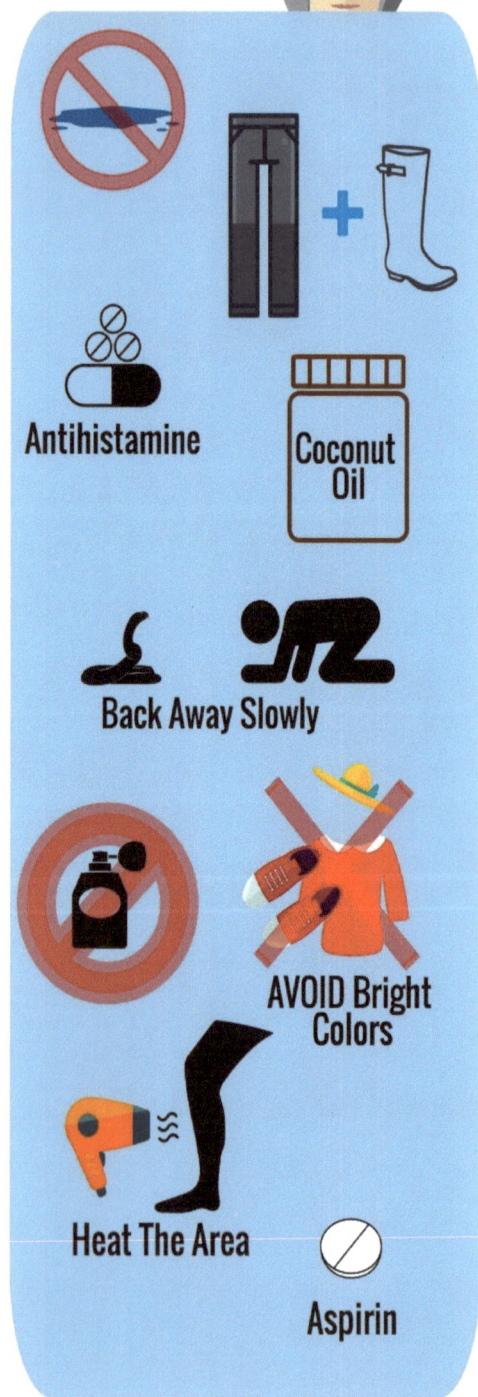

Bladder Infection

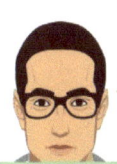
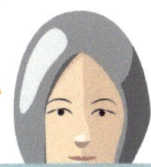

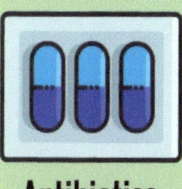
Antibiotics

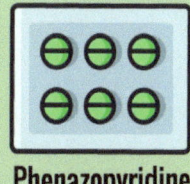
Phenazopyridine

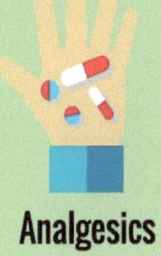
Analgesics

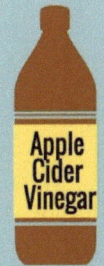
Apple Cider Vinegar

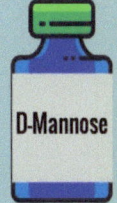
D-Mannose

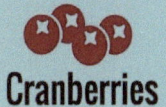
Cranberries

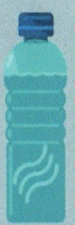

Blisters

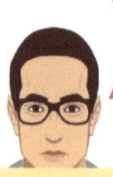
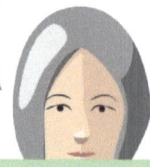

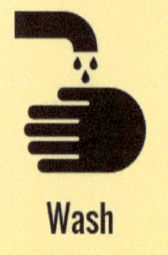
Wash

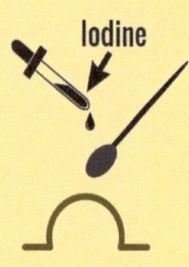
Iodine

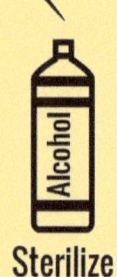
Sterilize

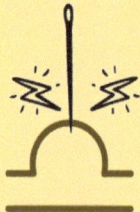
Puncture

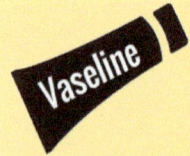
Vaseline

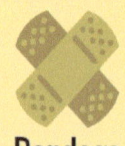
Bandage

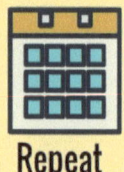
Repeat Daily

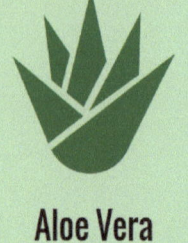
Aloe Vera

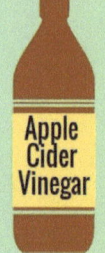
Apple Cider Vinegar

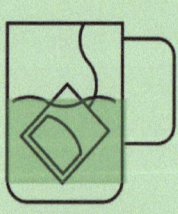
Green Tea

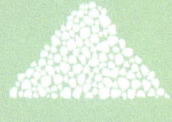
Epsom Salt

Blood Clots

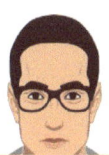 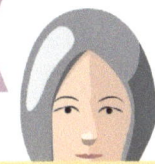

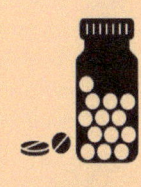
Aspirin

Anticoagulants
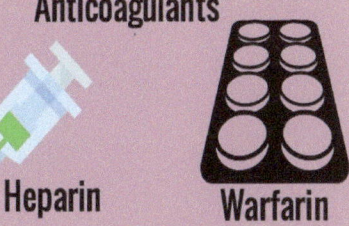
Heparin — Warfarin

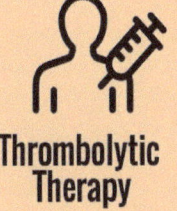
Thrombolytic Therapy

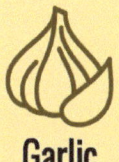
Garlic

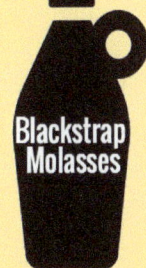
Blackstrap Molasses

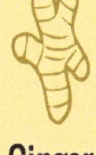
Ginger

Baking Soda

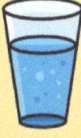

Body Odor

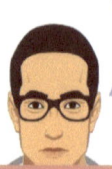
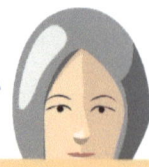
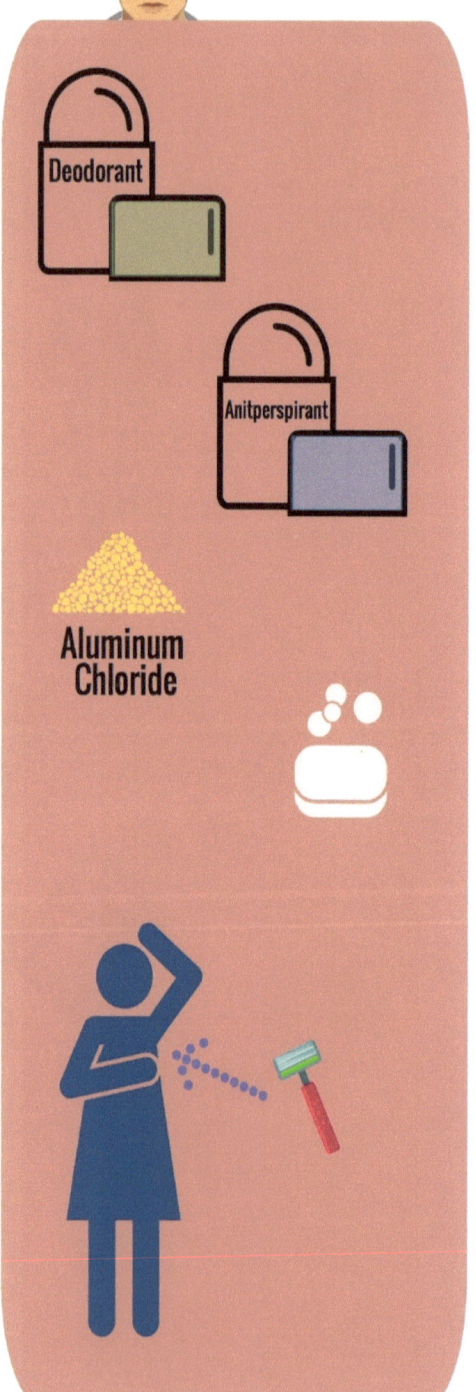

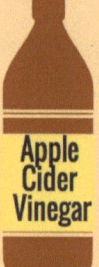
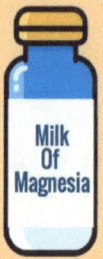
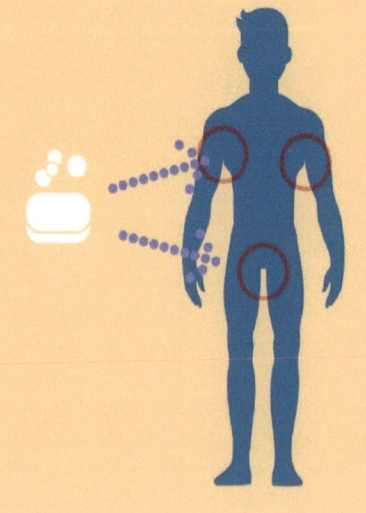

Boils

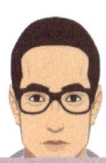
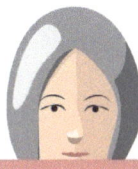

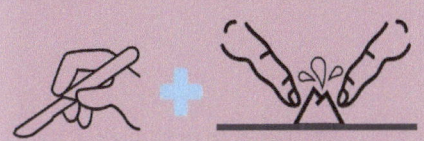
Incision + Drainage

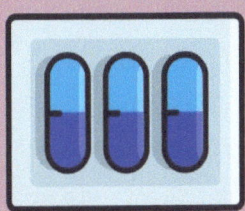
Antibiotics

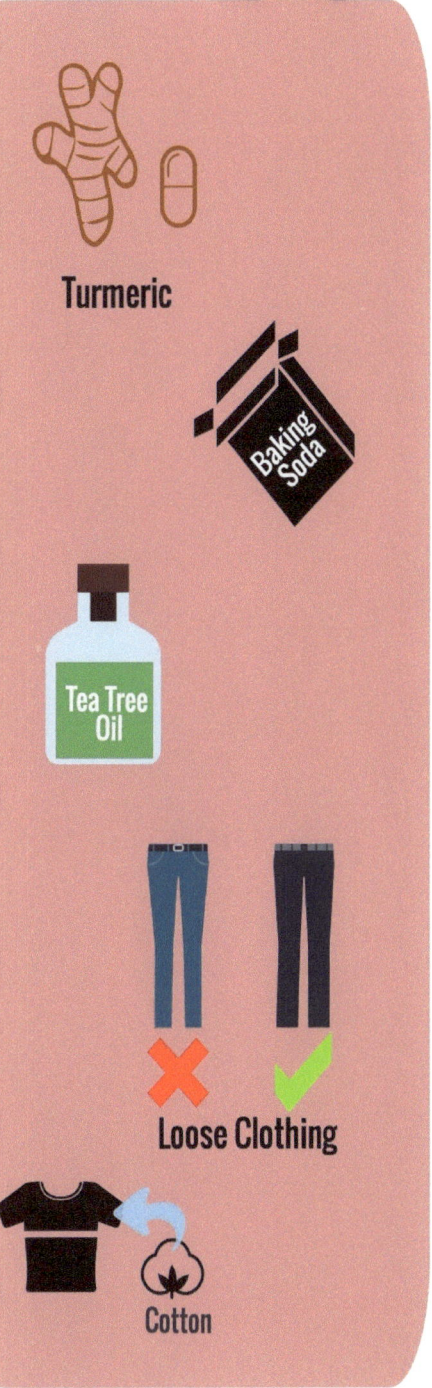

Turmeric

Tea Tree Oil

Loose Clothing

Cotton

Breast Cancer

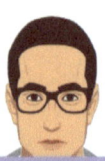 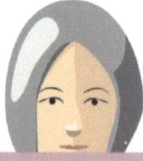

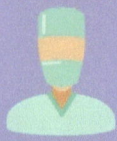
Surgery

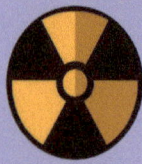
Radiation Therapy

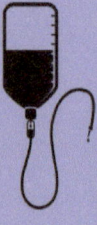
Chemotherapy

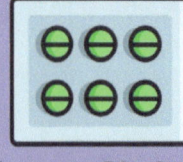
Hormone-Blocking Drugs

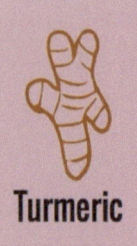
Turmeric

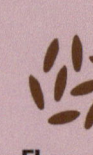
Flaxseed

 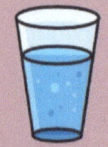

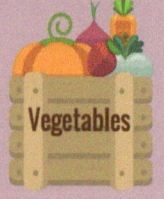
Vegetables

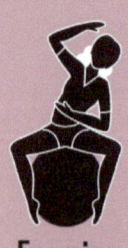
Exercise

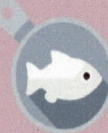

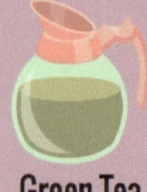
Green Tea

Breast Lumps

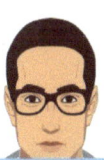
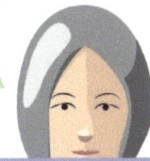

Wait

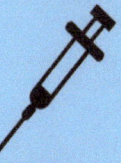
Needle Aspiration

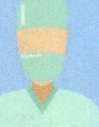
Surgery

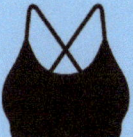
Athletic Bra

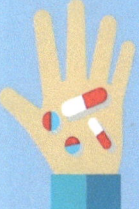
Pain Relievers

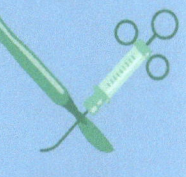
Biopsy

Evening Primrose Oil

Magnesium

Yoga

Apple Cider Vinegar

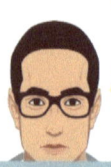 # Bronchitis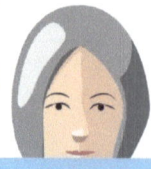

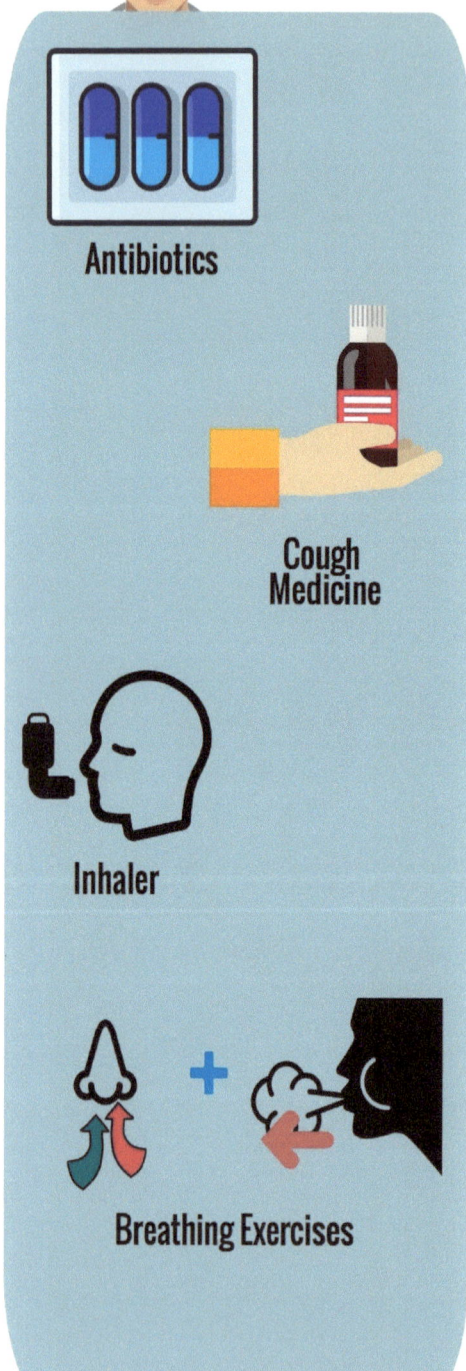
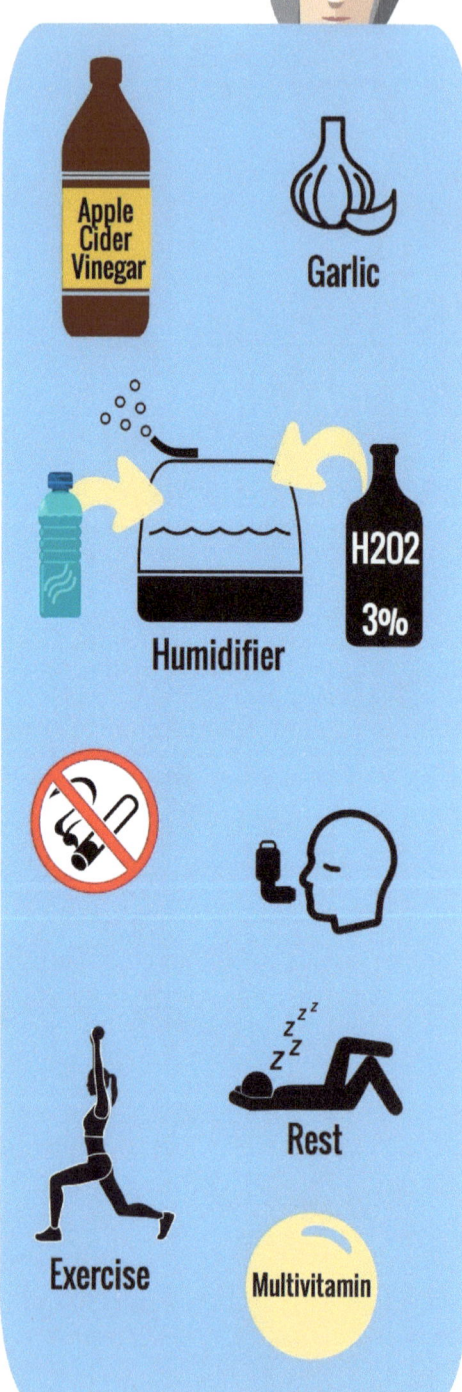

Bursitis

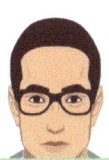
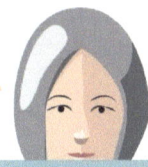
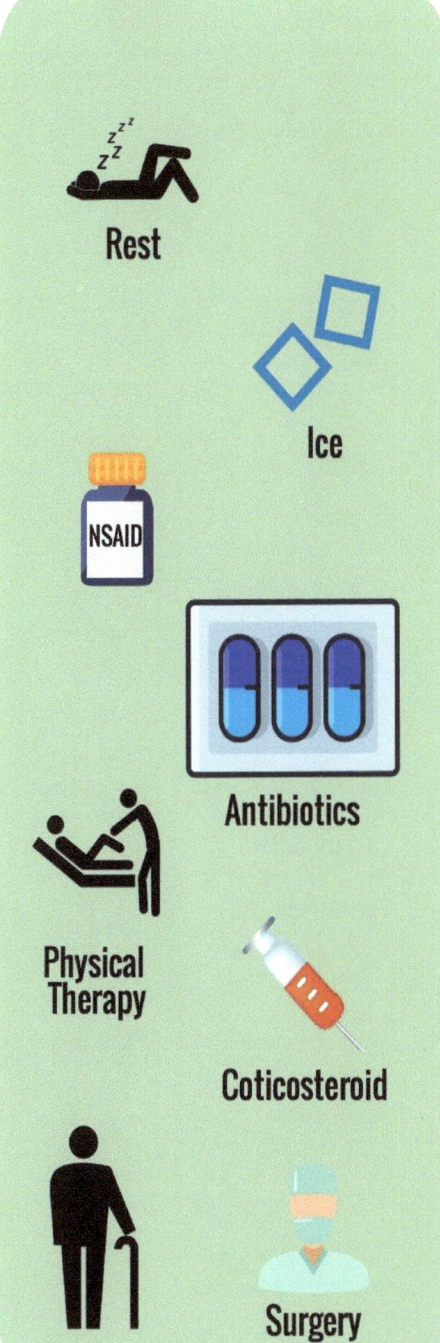

- Rest
- Ice
- NSAID
- Antibiotics
- Physical Therapy
- Coticosteroid
- Surgery

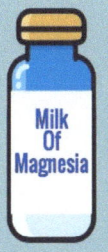 Milk Of Magnesia

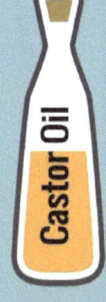 Castor Oil

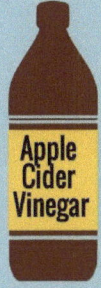 Apple Cider Vinegar

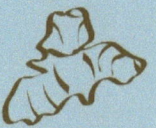 Ginger

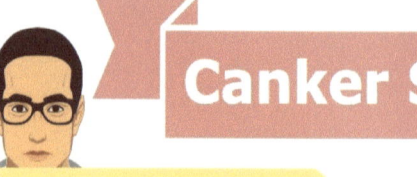
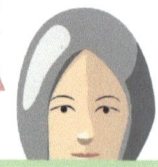

Canker Sores

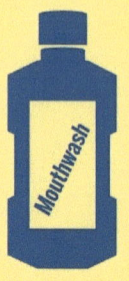
Mouthwash

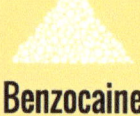
Benzocaine

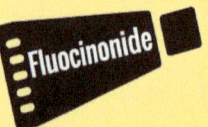
Fluocinonide

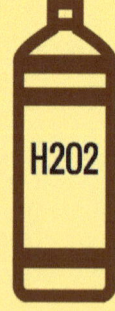
H2O2

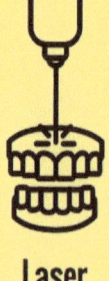
Laser

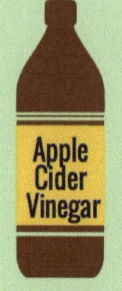
Apple Cider Vinegar

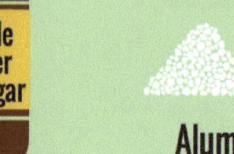
Alum

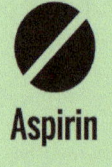
Aspirin

Baking Soda

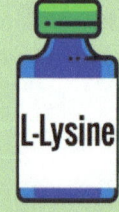
L-Lysine

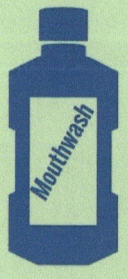
Mouthwash

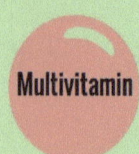
Multivitamin

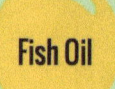
Fish Oil

Cataracts

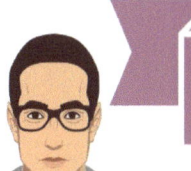
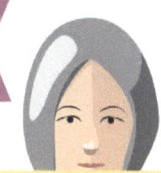

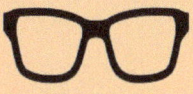
Eyeglasses

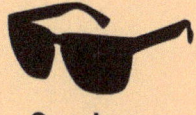
Sunglasses

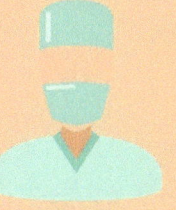
Surgery

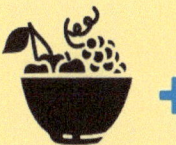 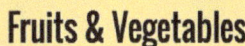
Fruits & Vegetables

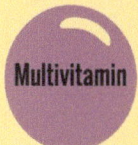
Multivitamin

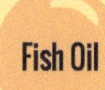
Fish Oil

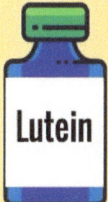
Lutein

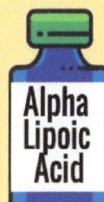
Alpha Lipoic Acid

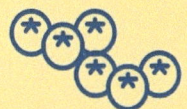
Bilberry Extract

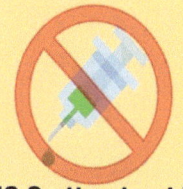
NO Corticosteroid

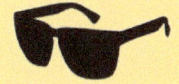

Cavities

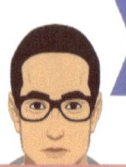
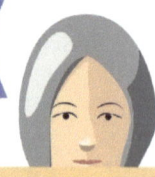

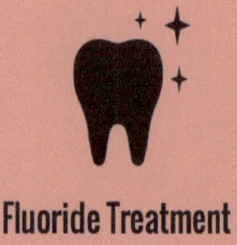
Fluoride Treatment

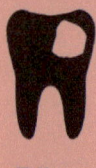
Filling

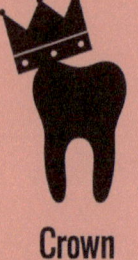
Crown

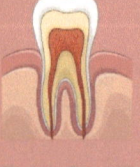
Root Canal

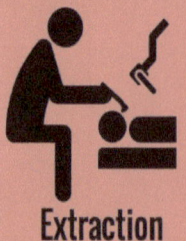
Extraction

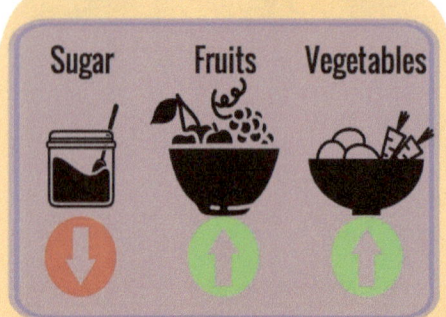
Sugar | Fruits | Vegetables

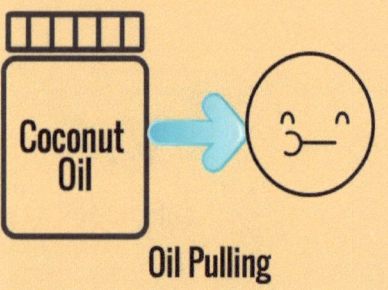
Oil Pulling

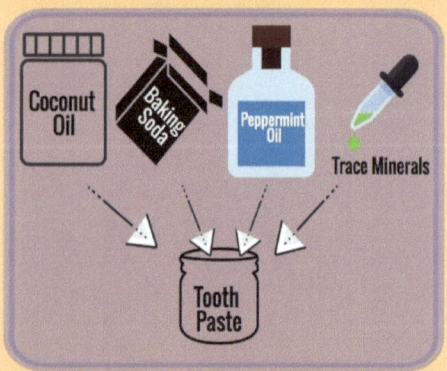

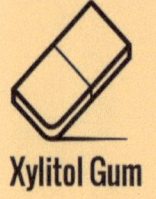
Xylitol Gum

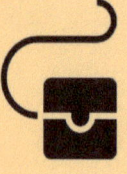

Cervical Dysplasia

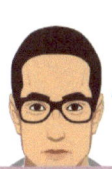
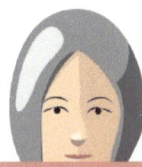

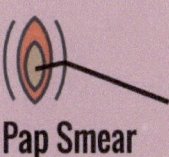
Pap Smear

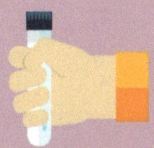
HPV Test

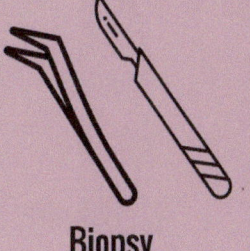
Biopsy

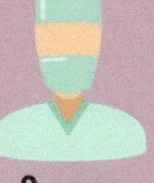
Surgery

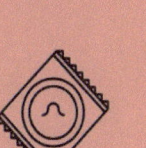
Pap Smear

Condoms

Vegetables

Multivitamin

Fish Oil

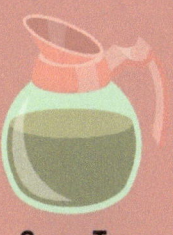
Green Tea Extract

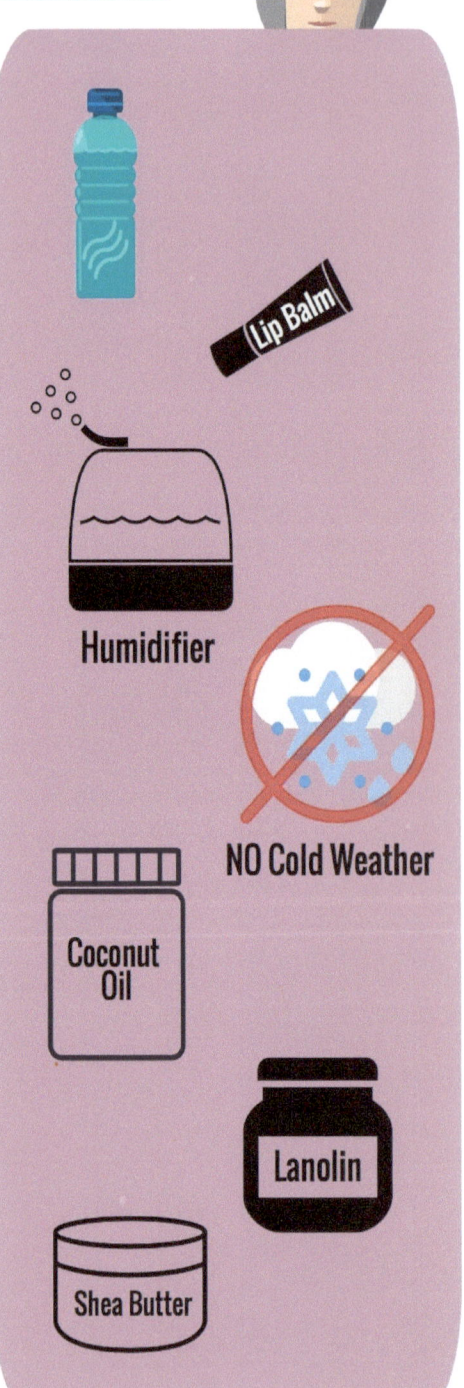

Chapped Lips

- Lip Balm Sunscreen
- AVOID Licking Lips
- Breathe Through Nose
- Humidifier
- NO Cold Weather
- Coconut Oil
- Lanolin
- Shea Butter
- Lip Balm

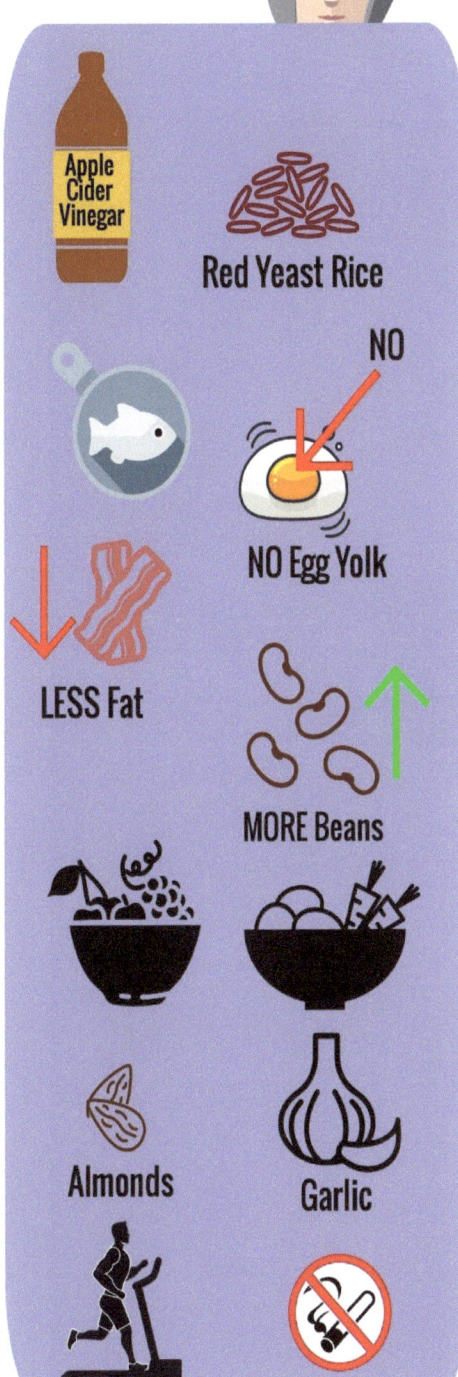

Cold Hands & Feet (Circulation)

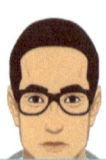 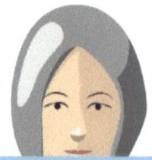

Pentoxifylline

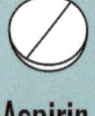
Aspirin

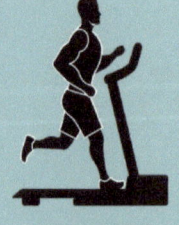
Exercise

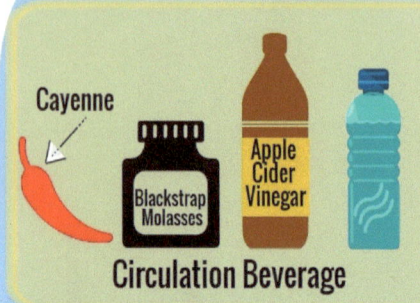
Cayenne · Blackstrap Molasses · Apple Cider Vinegar
Circulation Beverage

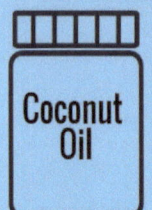
Coconut Oil

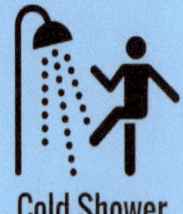
Cold Shower

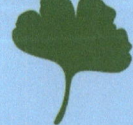
Ginko Biloba

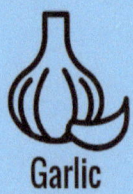
Garlic

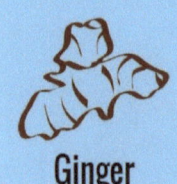
Ginger

Cold

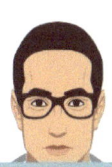
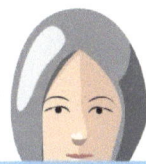

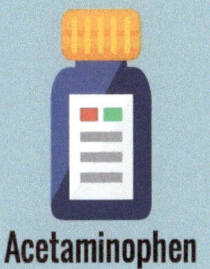
Acetaminophen

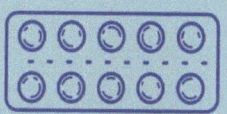
Decongestant

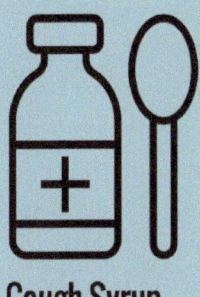
Cough Syrup

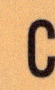

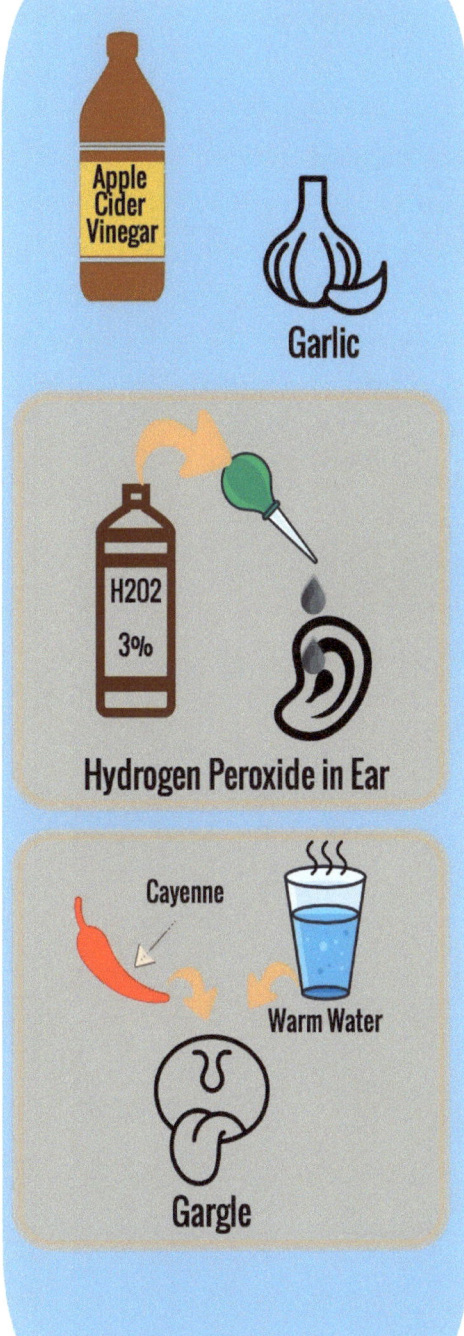

Cold Sores
Acyclovir
Valacyclovir
Cold Sore Cream
Lip Balm Sunscreen
Lidocaine
Benzocaine
Acetone
H2O2 3%
Apple Cider Vinegar
L-Lysine
Ear Wax
C

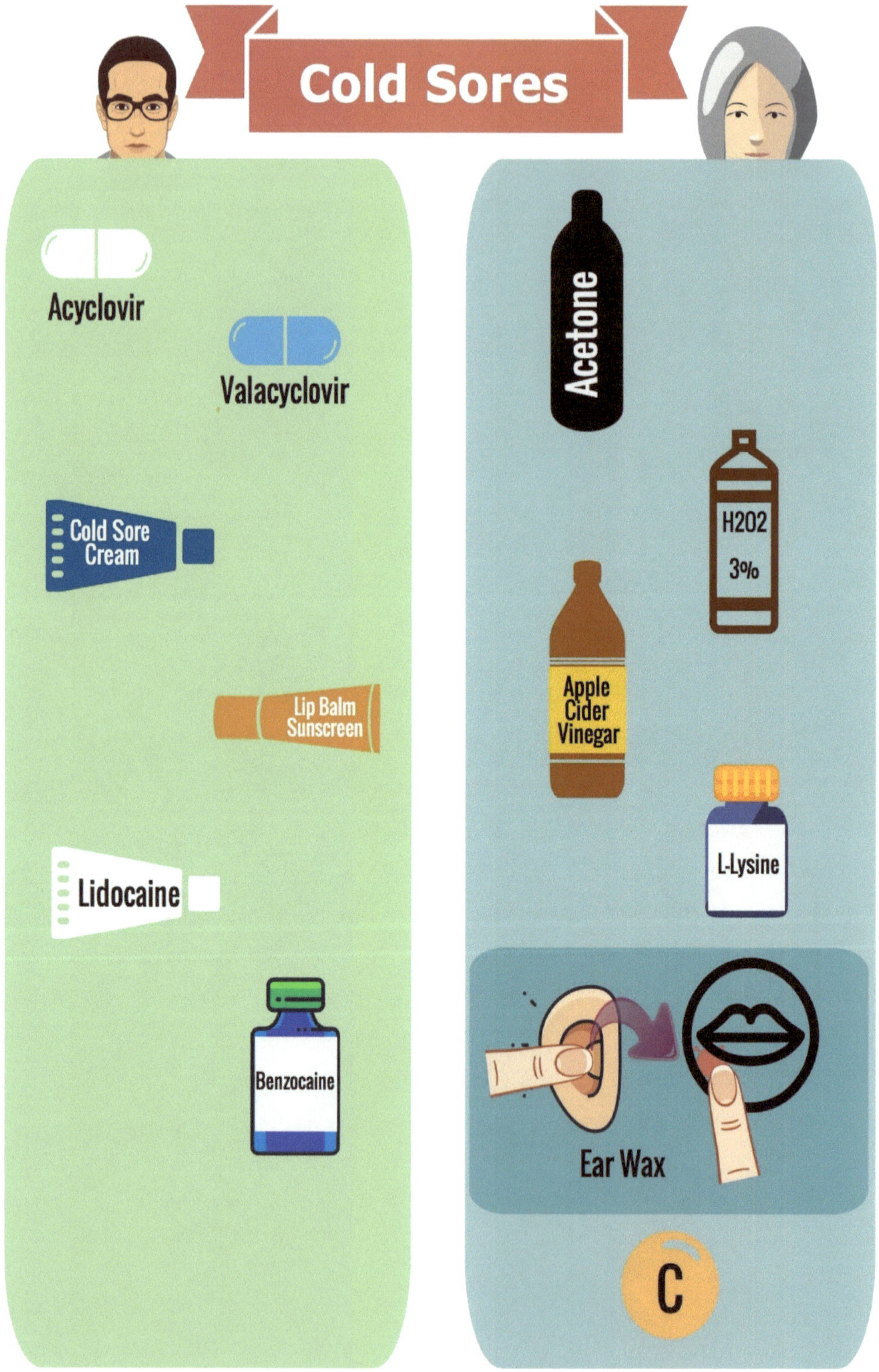

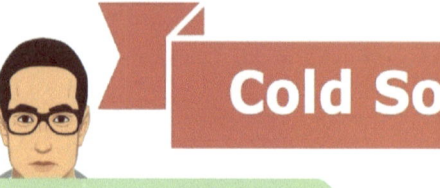

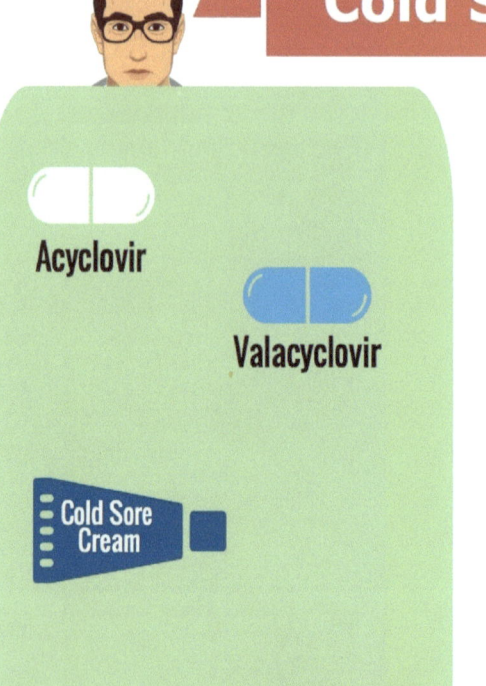

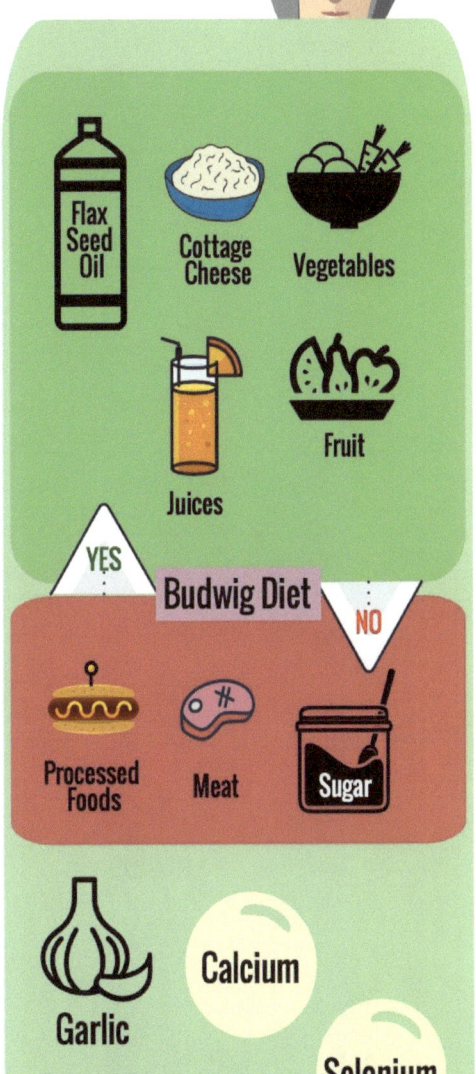

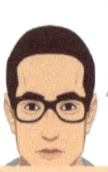 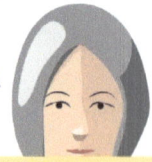

Constipation

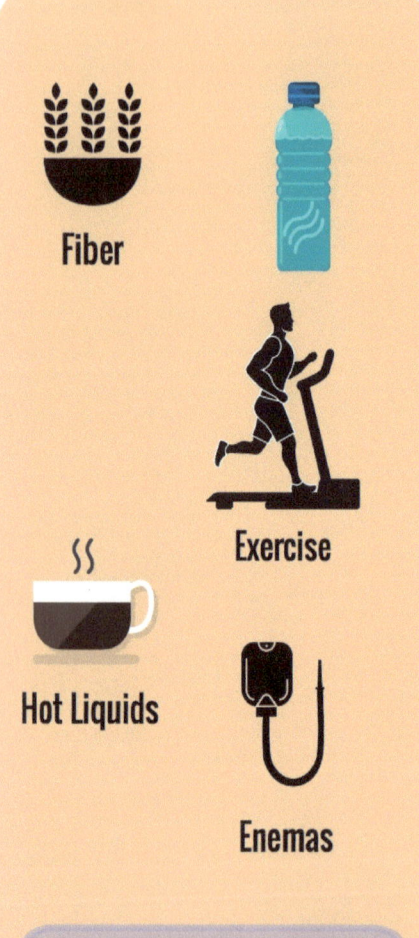
- Fiber
- Hot Liquids
- Exercise
- Enemas
- Laxatives

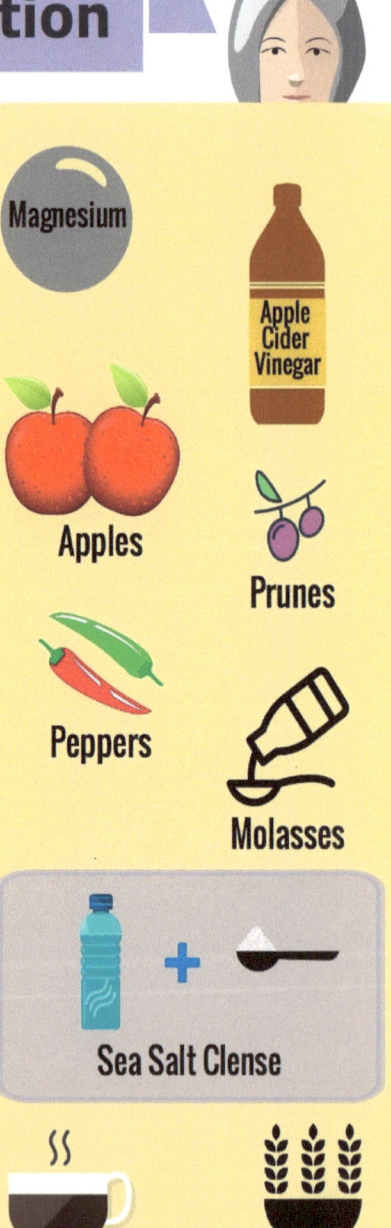
- Magnesium
- Apple Cider Vinegar
- Apples
- Prunes
- Peppers
- Molasses
- Sea Salt Clense
- Hot Liquids
- Fiber

Calluses (Corns)

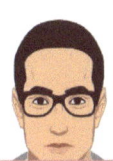
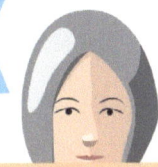

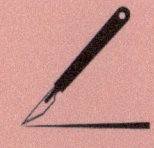
Cut Excess Skin

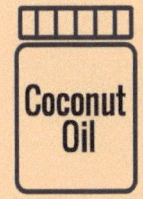
Coconut Oil

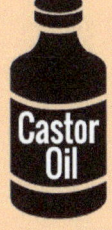
Castor Oil

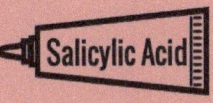
Salicylic Acid

Baking Soda

Pumice Stone

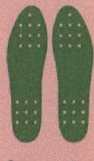
Antibiotic

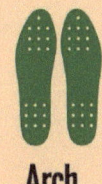
Arch Support

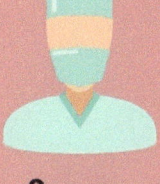
Inserts

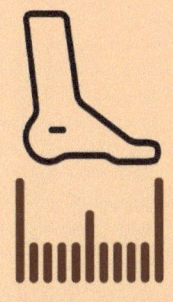
Get Measured

Surgery

Cough

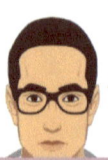
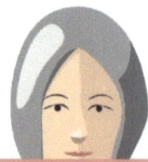

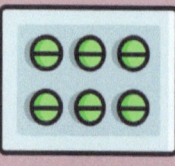
Antibiotics

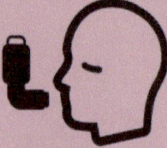
Inhaler

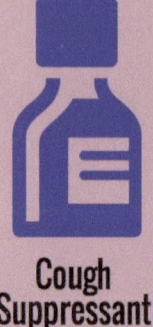
Cough Suppressant

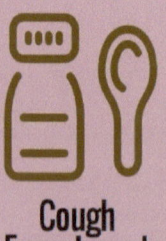
Cough Expectorant

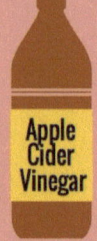
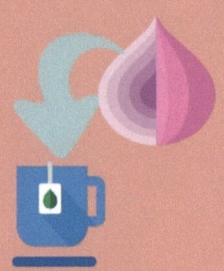
Onion Tea

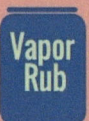
Vapor Rub

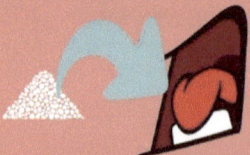
Sea Salt Gargle

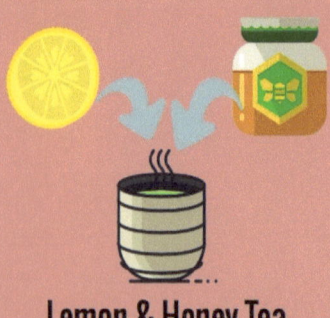
Lemon & Honey Tea

Dandruff

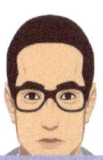
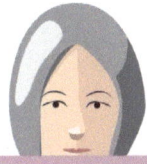

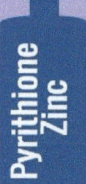 Pyrithione Zinc

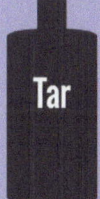 Tar

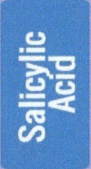 Salicylic Acid

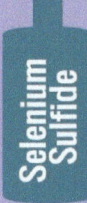 Selenium Sulfide

Ketoconazole

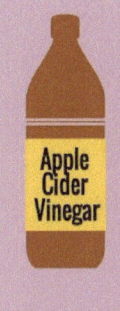 Apple Cider Vinegar

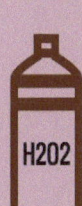 H2O2

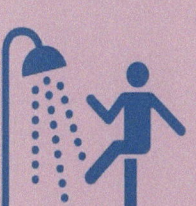
Cold Shower

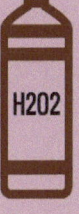 Tea Tree Oil

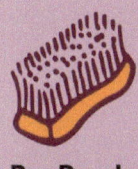
Dry Brush Massage

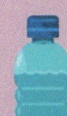

NO Hats

Depression

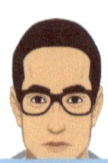 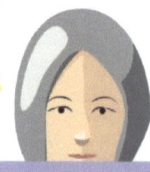

- Antidepressants
- Psychotherapy
- Electroconvulsive Therapy
- Transcranial Magnetic Stimulation

- Apple Cider Vinegar
- Cold Shower
- Fish Oil
- 5 HTP
- St John's Wort
- Exercise
- Reduce Stress
- Multivitamin
- NO Aspartame
- Sun

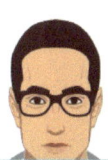 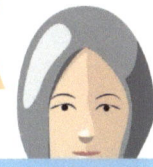

Dermatitis (Eczema)

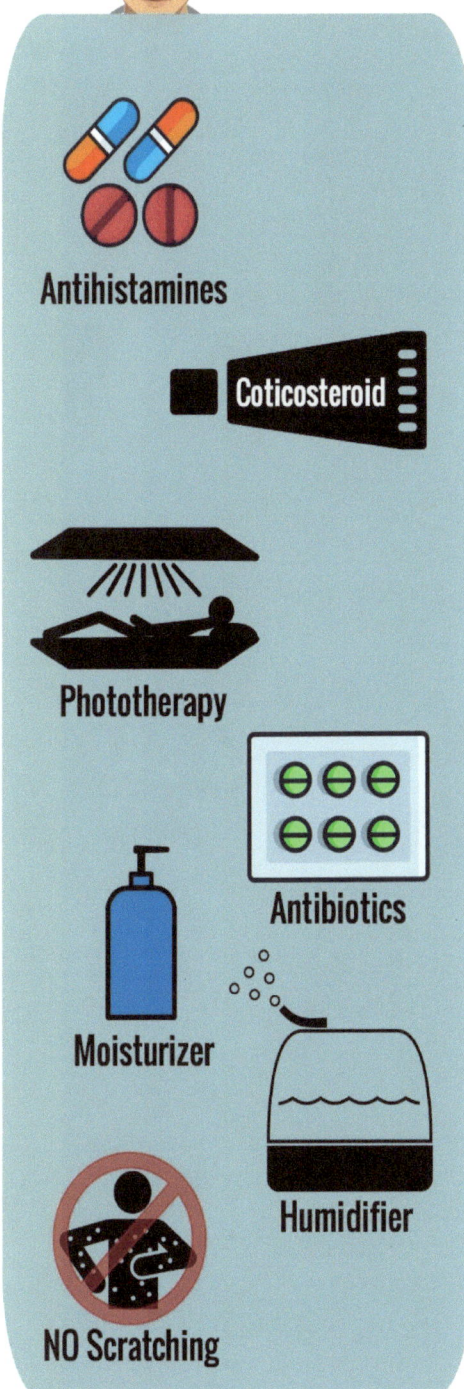
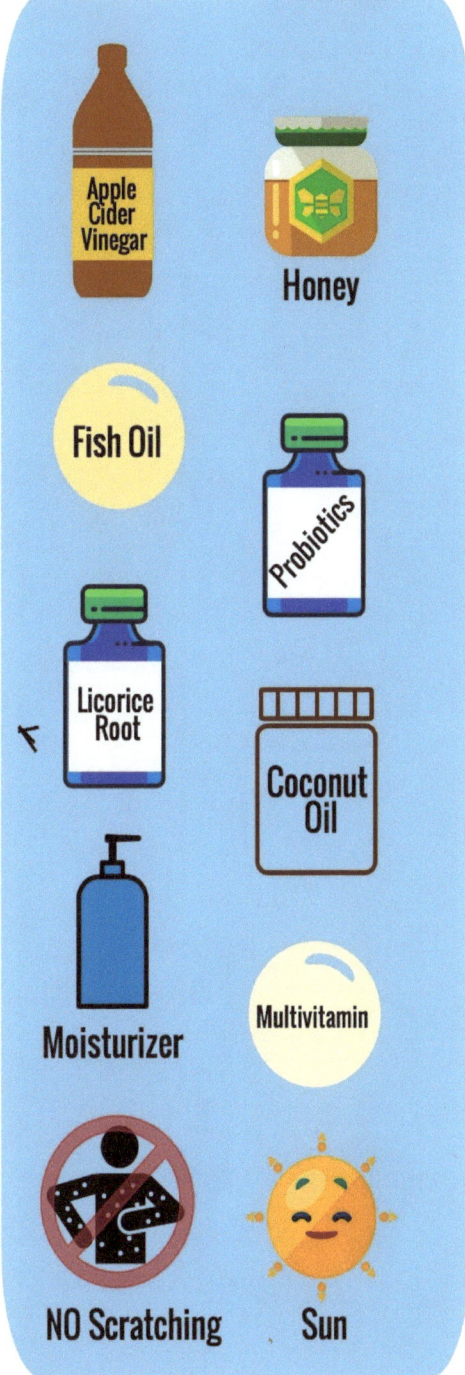

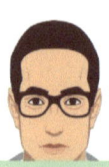 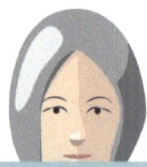

Diabetes

- Insulin
- Blood Sugar Monitoring (105)
- Healthy Food
- Exercise
- Lose Weight

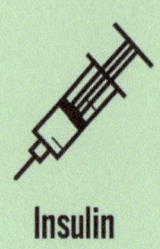
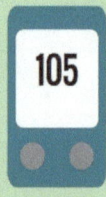
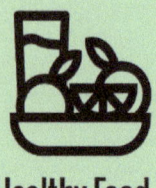
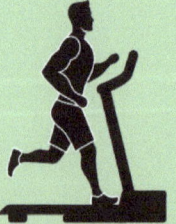
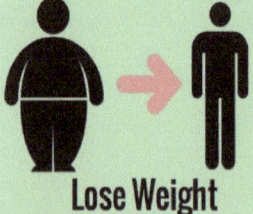

- Apple Cider Vinegar
- Lose Weight
- Multivitamin
- Exercise
- Sugar ↓
- Fruit ↑
- Fish ↑
- Vegetables ↑

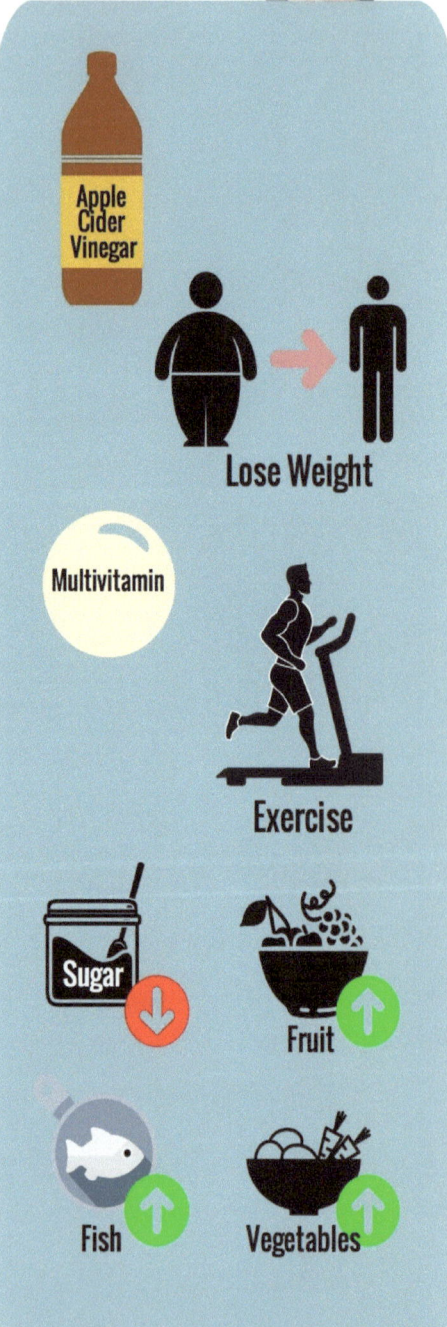

Diarrhea

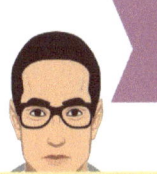
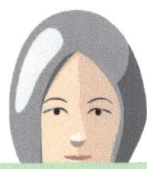

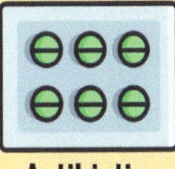
Antibiotics

Liquids

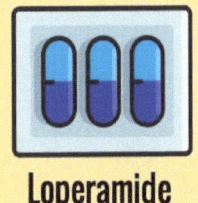
Loperamide

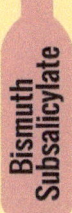
Bismuth Subsalicylate

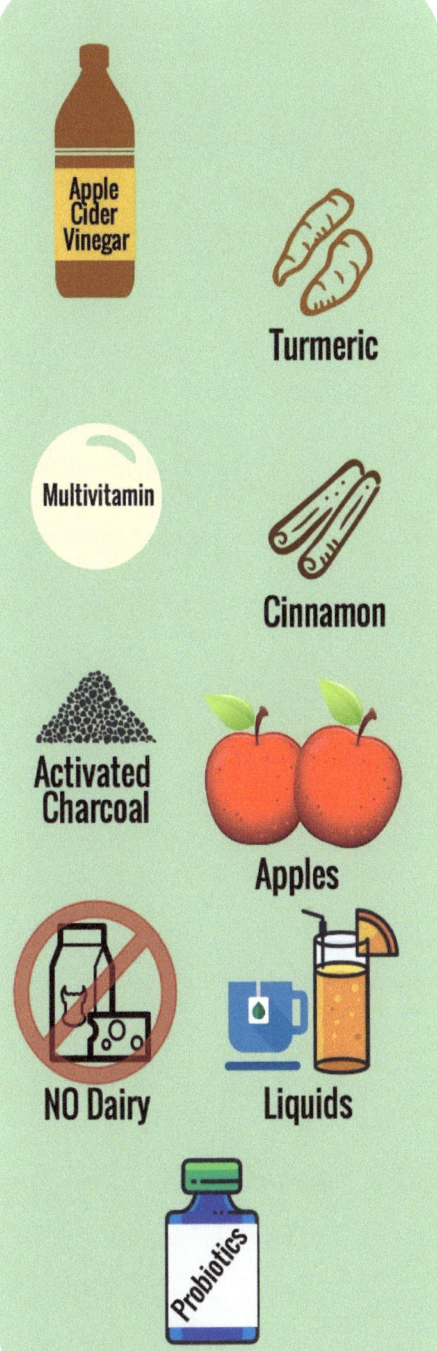

Apple Cider Vinegar

Turmeric

Multivitamin

Cinnamon

Activated Charcoal

Apples

NO Dairy

Liquids

Probiotics

Diverticulosis

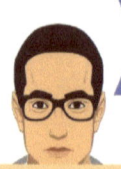
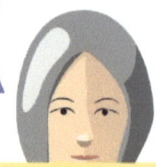

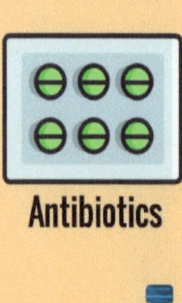
Antibiotics

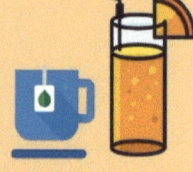
Liquid Diet

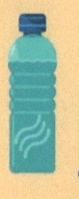
Acetaminophen

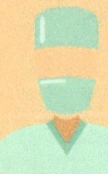
Surgery

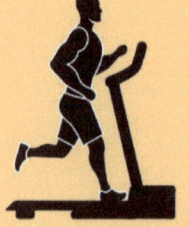
Exercise

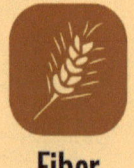
Fiber

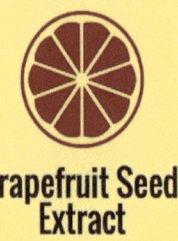
Grapefruit Seed Extract

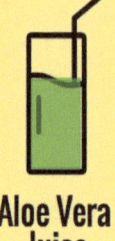
Aloe Vera Juice

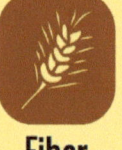
Fiber

Fruits & Vegetables

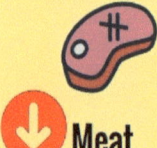
↓ Meat

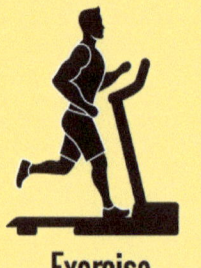
Exercise

Dizziness

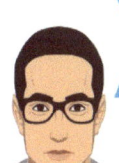
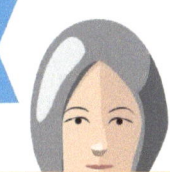

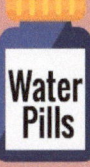
Water Pills

Antihistamine

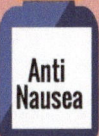
Anti Nausea

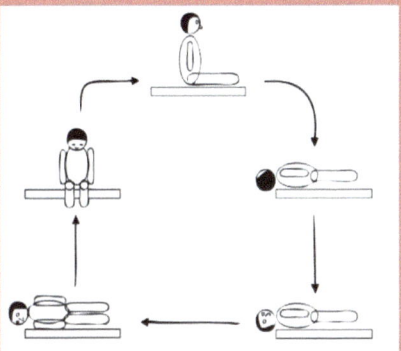
Epley Maneuver

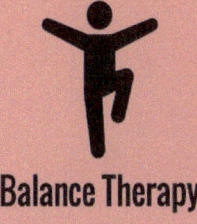
Balance Therapy

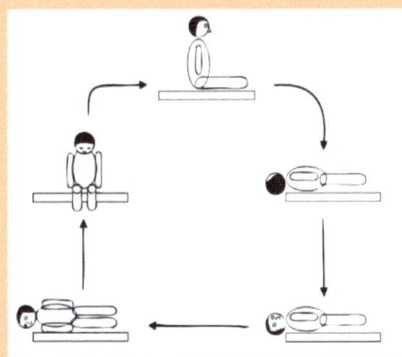
Epley Maneuver

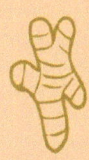
Ginger

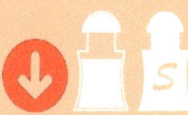
Less Salt

Don't Read In Vehicle

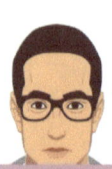 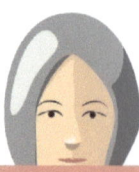

Dry Hair

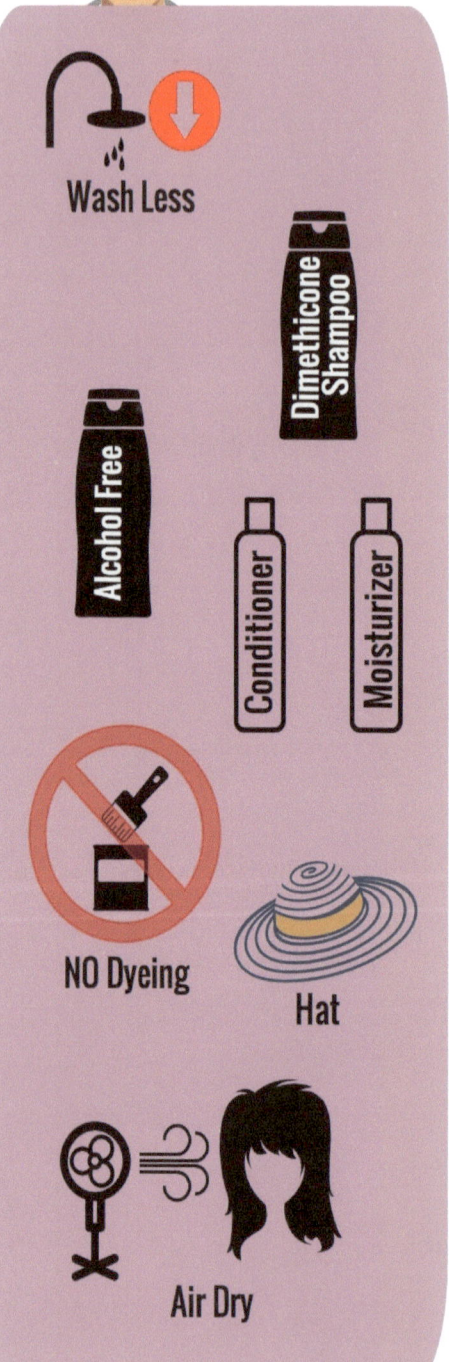 

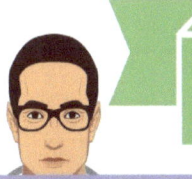 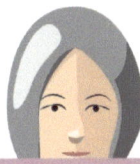

Dry Eyes

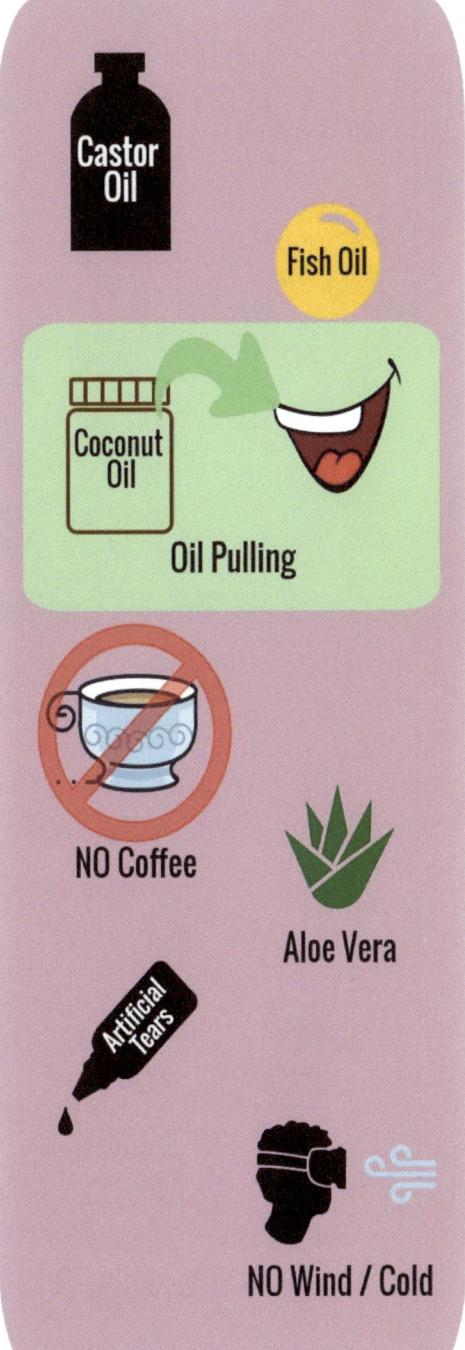

- Antibiotics
- Artificial Tears Insert
- Scleral Contact Lenses
- Light Therapy
- Eye Massage

- Castor Oil
- Fish Oil
- Oil Pulling (Coconut Oil)
- NO Coffee
- Aloe Vera
- Artificial Tears
- NO Wind / Cold

Dry Mouth

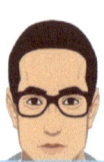
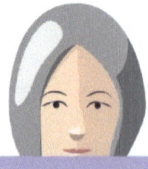
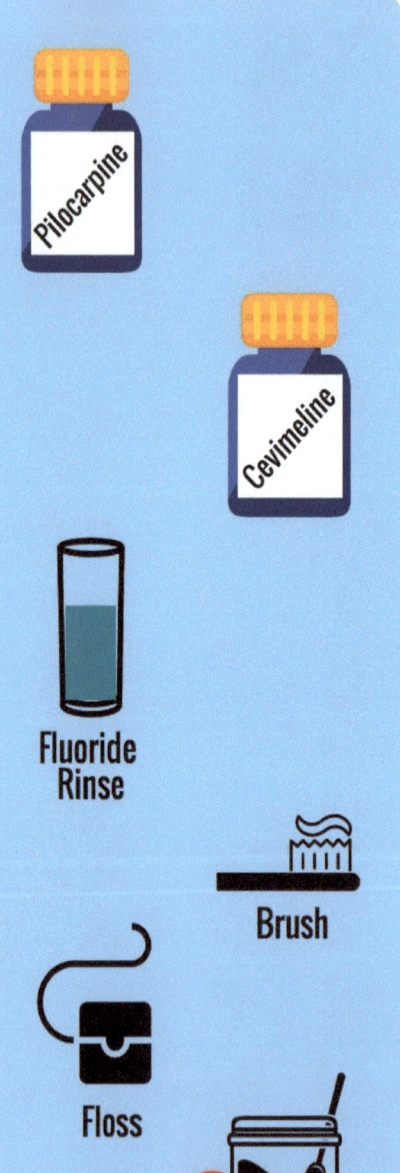
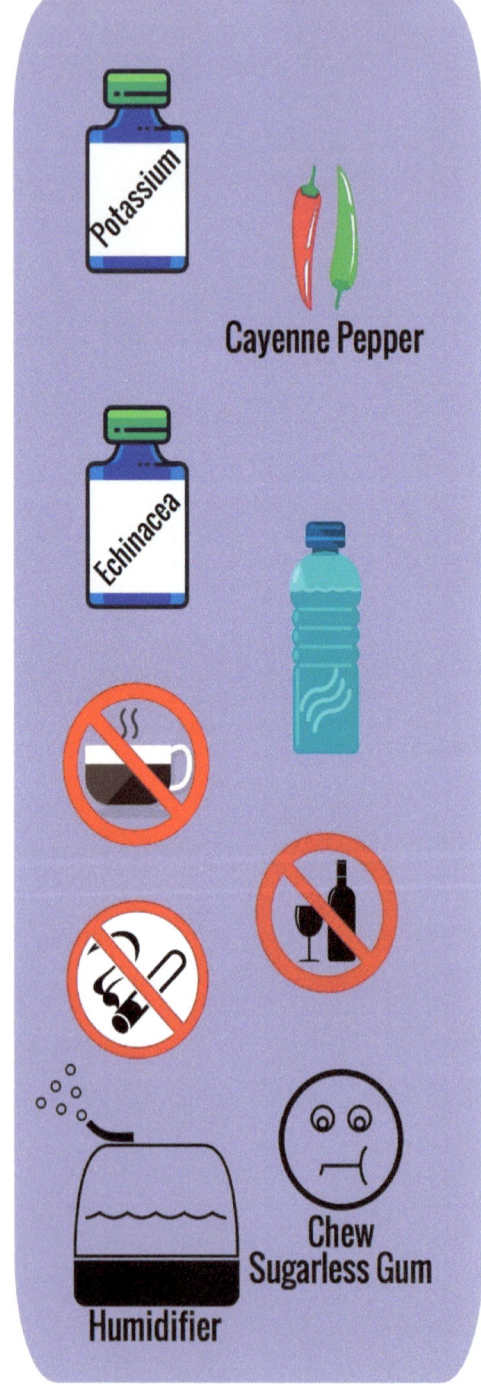

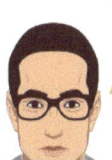 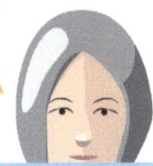

Dry Skin

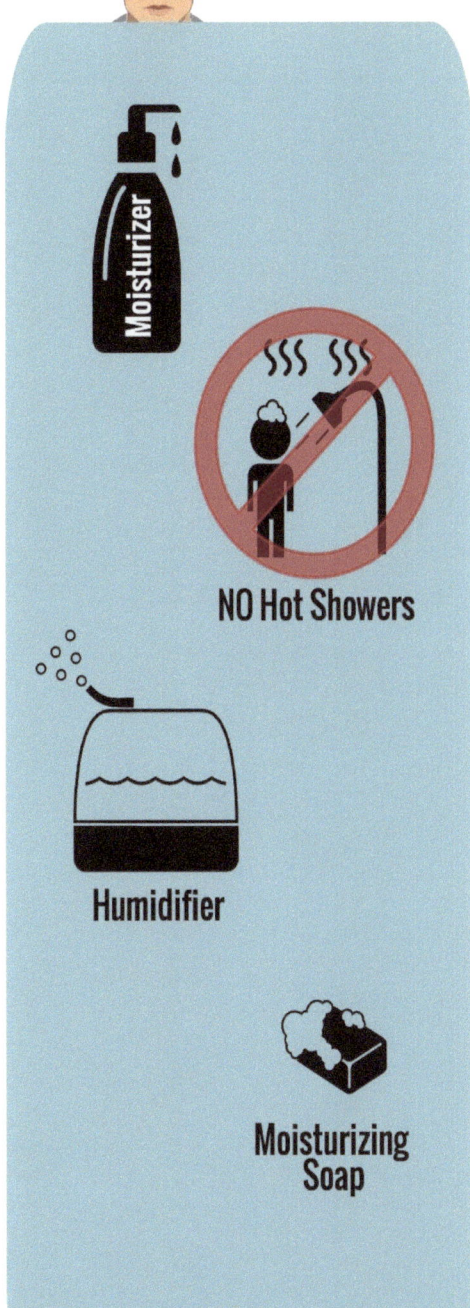

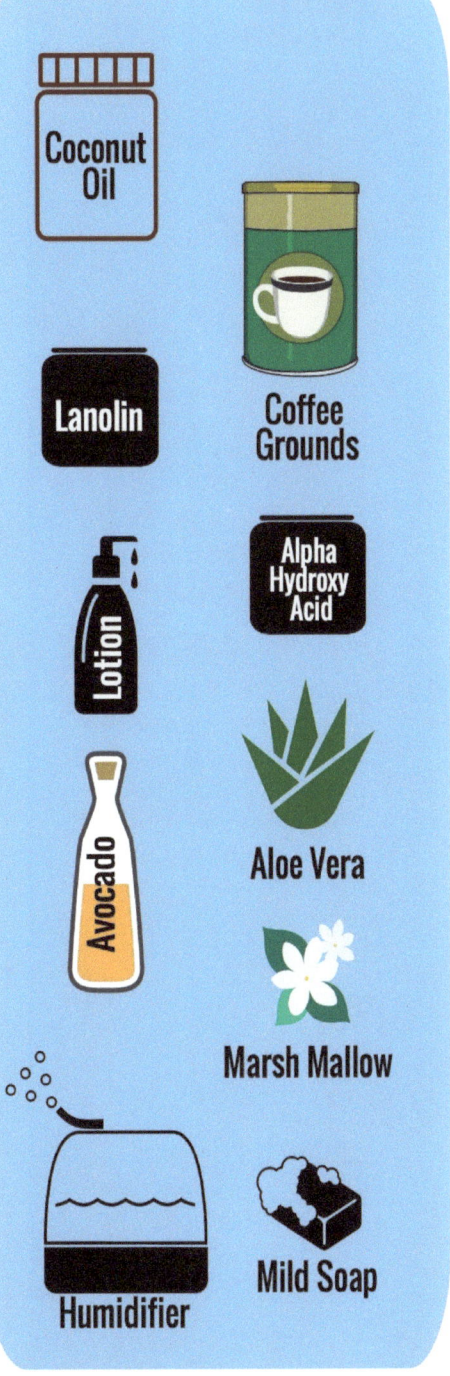

Ear Ache

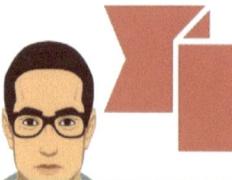
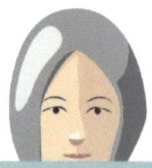
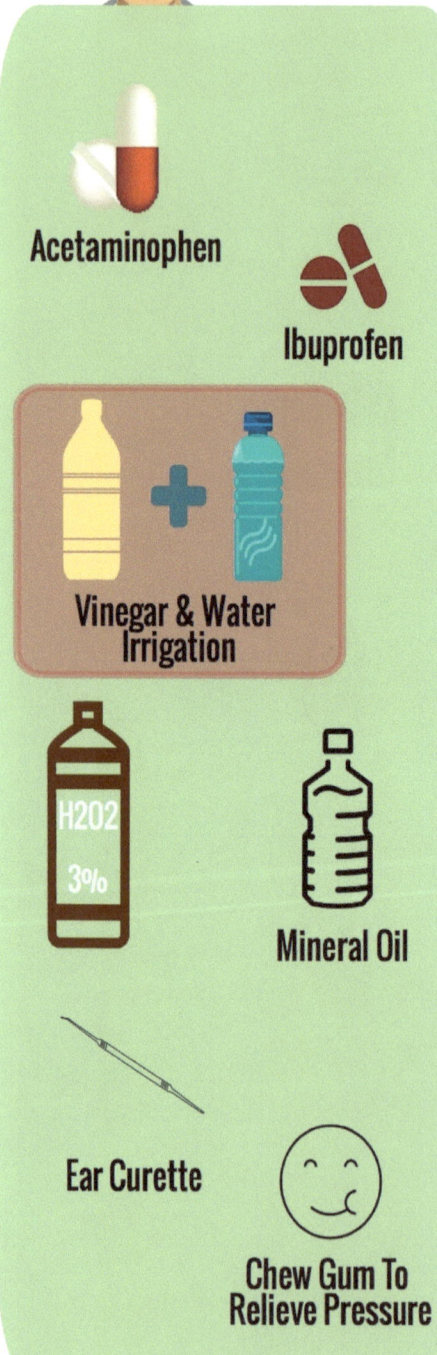
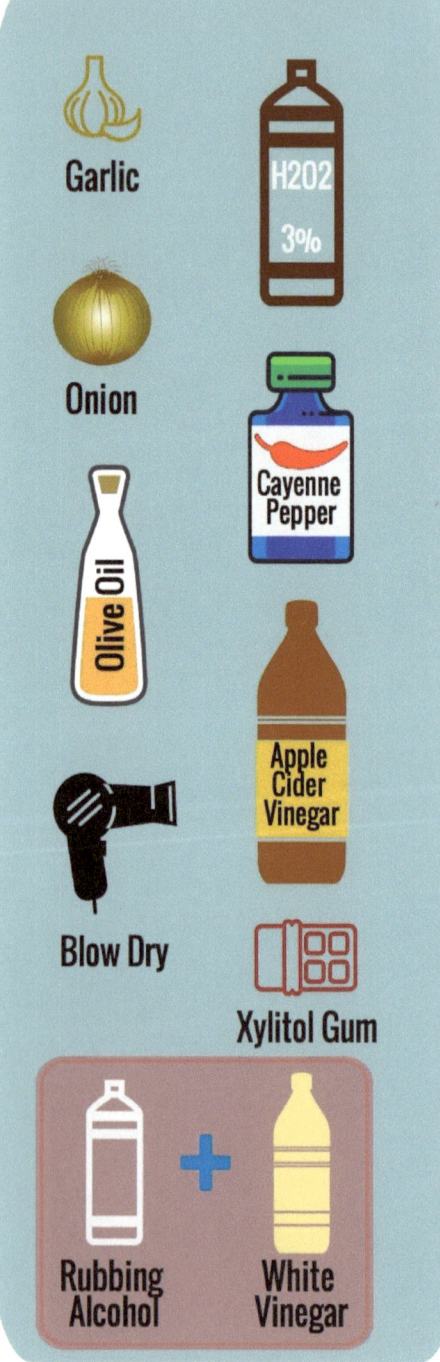

Erectile Dysfunction

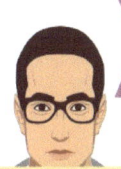
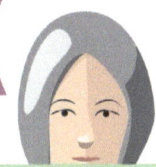
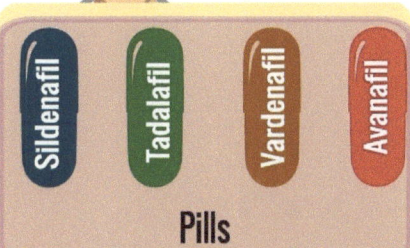
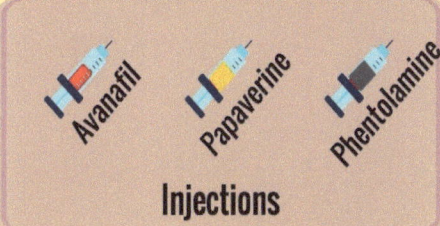
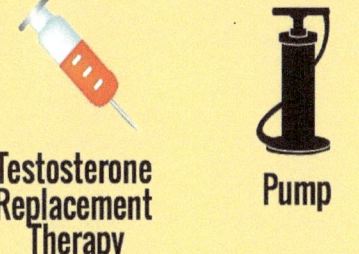
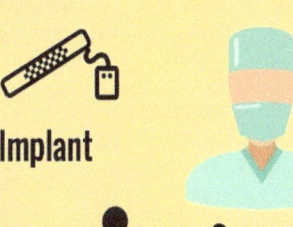
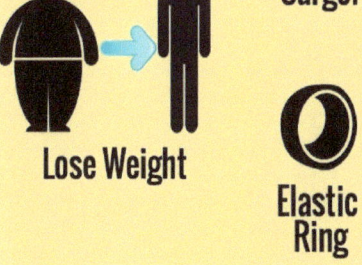
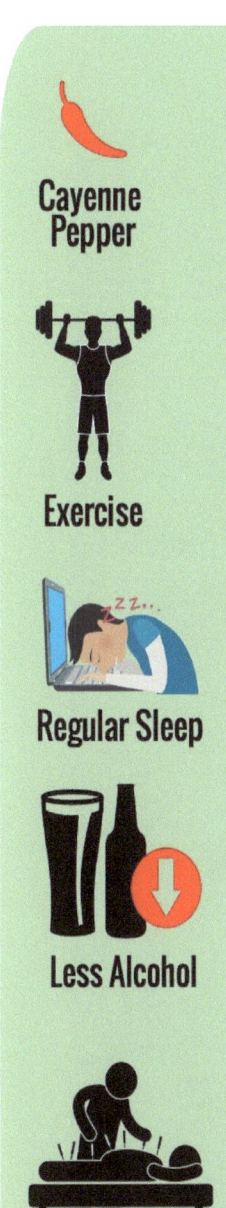
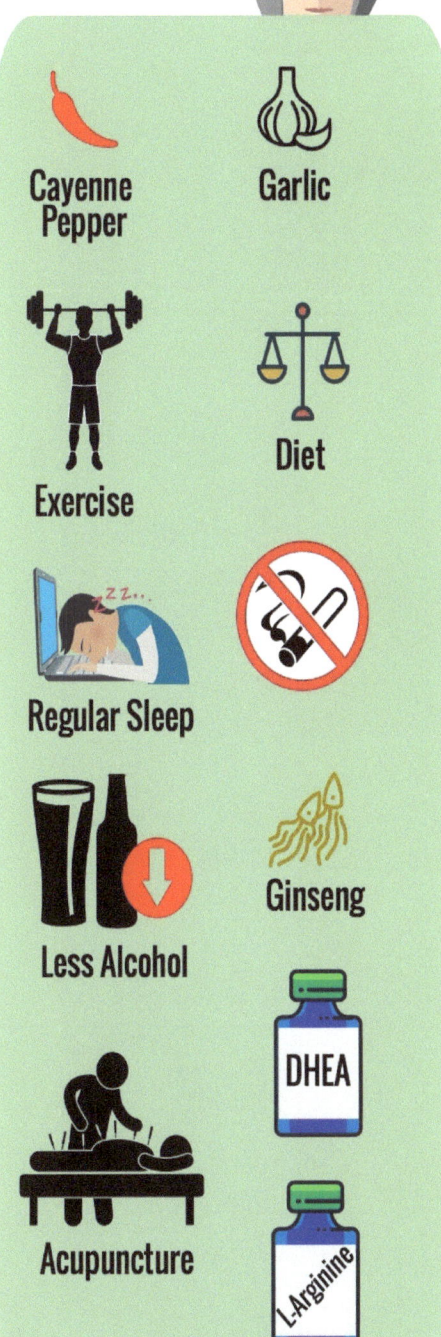

Fatigue

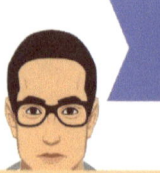
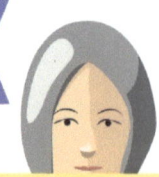

NO Alcohol

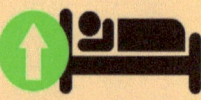
More Sleep

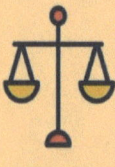
Diet

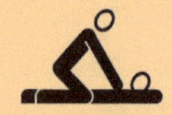
Physical Therapy

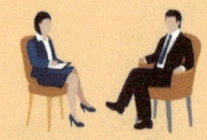
Cognitive Behavioral Therapy

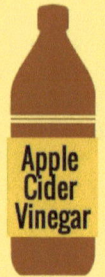
Apple Cider Vinegar

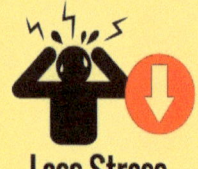
Less Stress

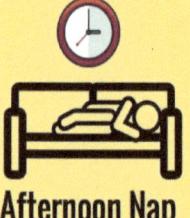
Afternoon Nap

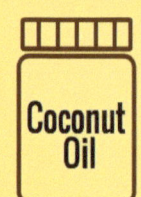
Coconut Oil

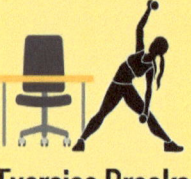
Exercise Breaks

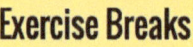

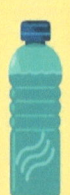

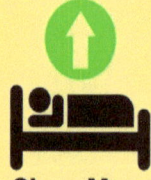
Sleep More

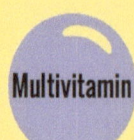
Multivitamin

Flatulence

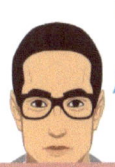
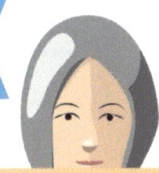

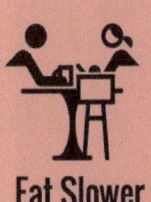
Eat Slower

NO Gum Chewing

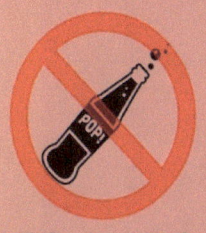
NO Carbonated Beverages

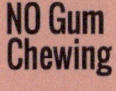
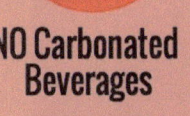
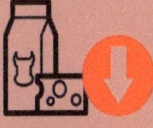

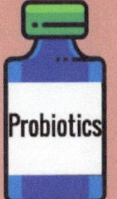
Probiotics

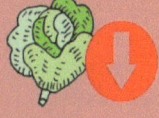

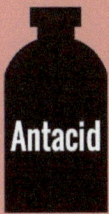
Antacid

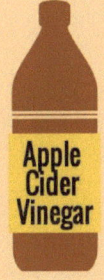
Apple Cider Vinegar

Baking Soda

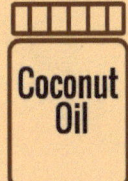
Coconut Oil

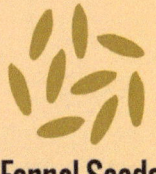
Fennel Seeds

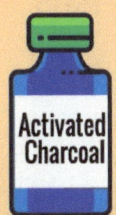
Activated Charcoal

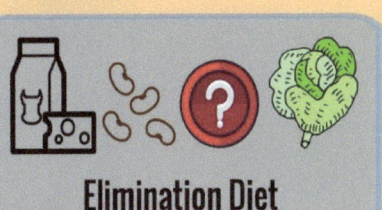
Elimination Diet

Flu

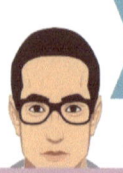
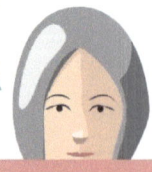
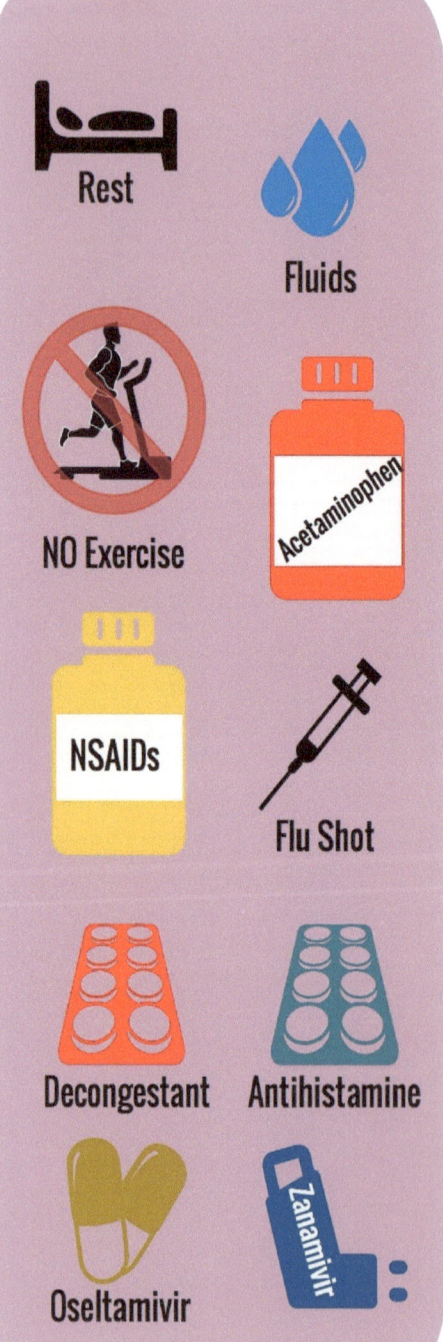
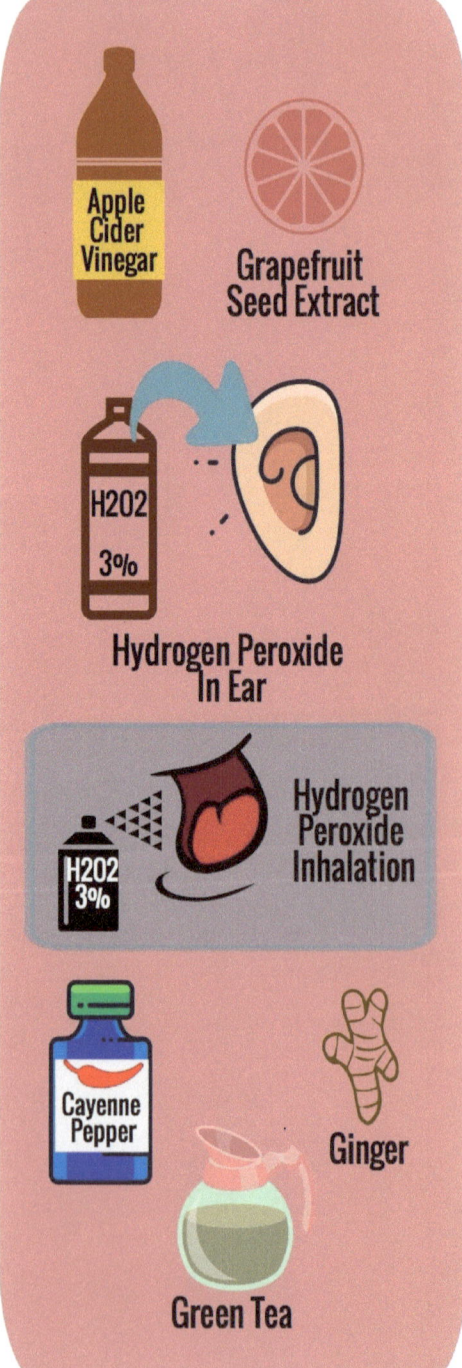

Food Allergies

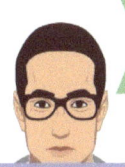
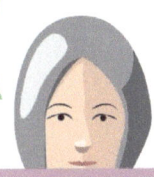
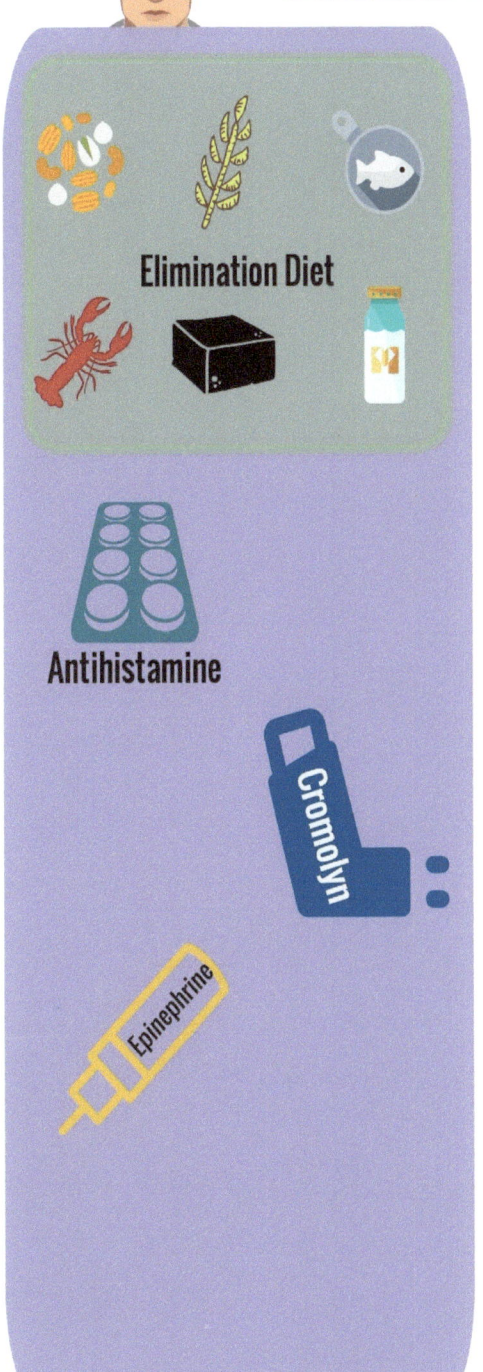
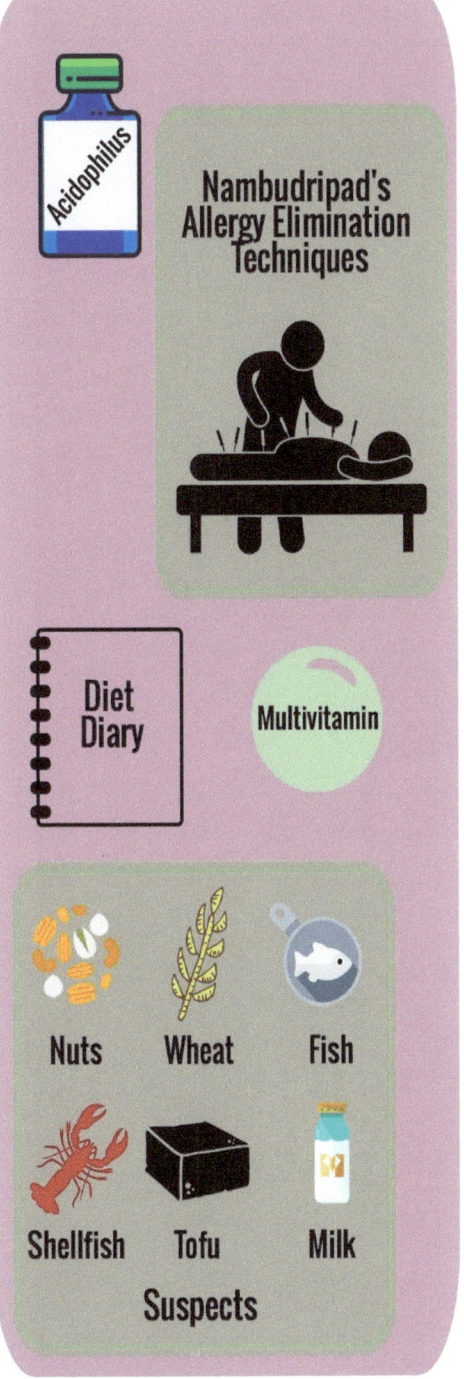

Food Poisoning

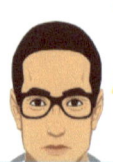
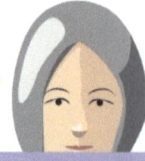

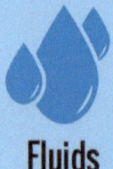
Fluids

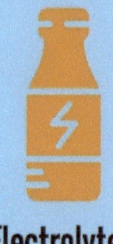
Electrolytes

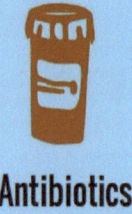
Antibiotics

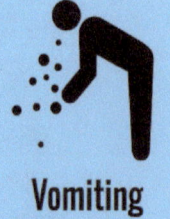
Vomiting

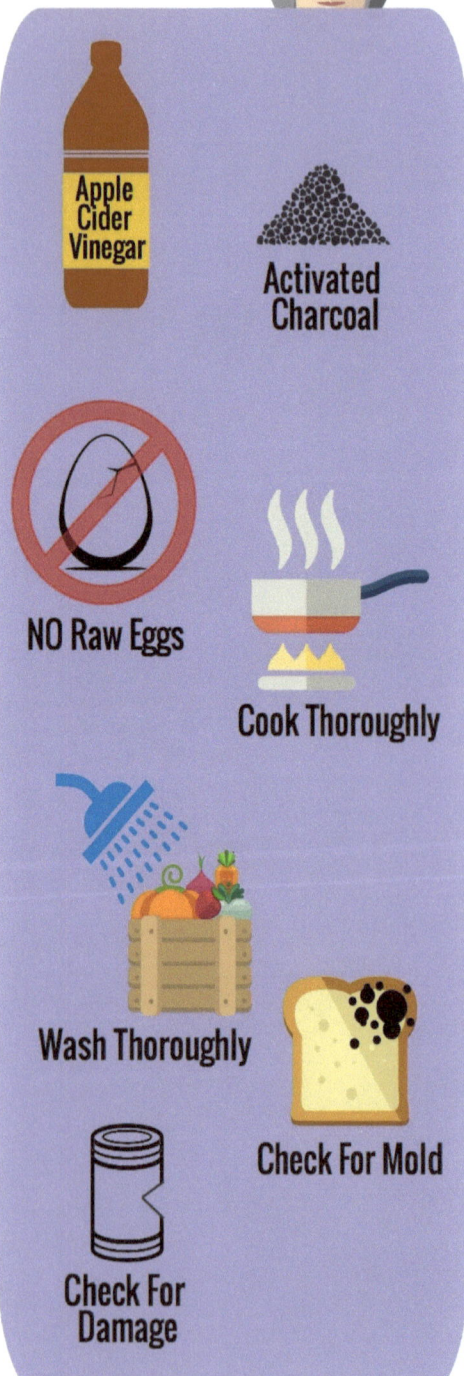

Apple Cider Vinegar

Activated Charcoal

NO Raw Eggs

Cook Thoroughly

Wash Thoroughly

Check For Mold

Check For Damage

Foot Odor

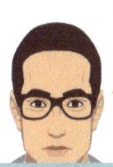
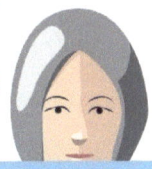

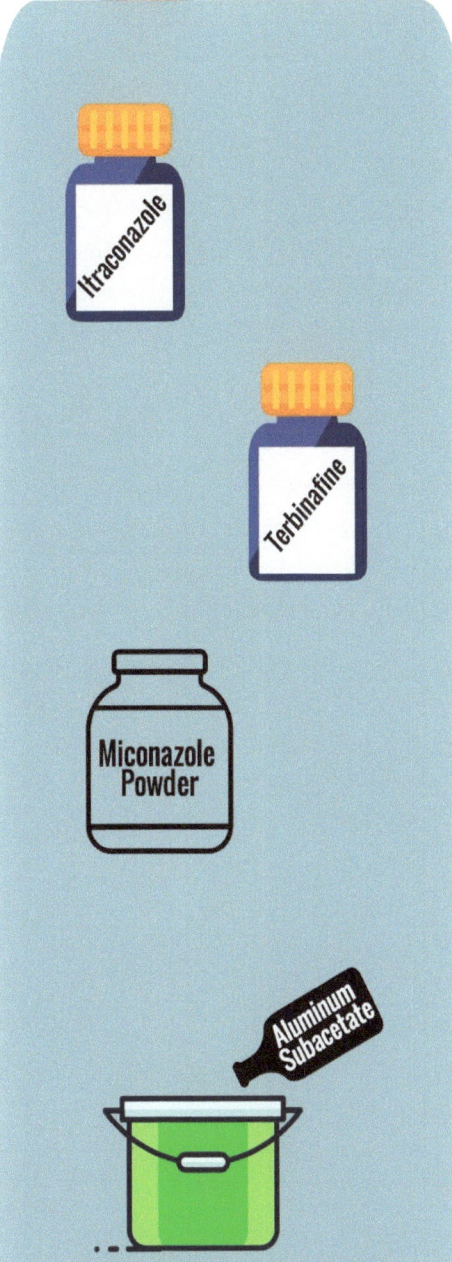

- Itraconazole
- Terbinafine
- Miconazole Powder
- Aluminum Subacetate Soak

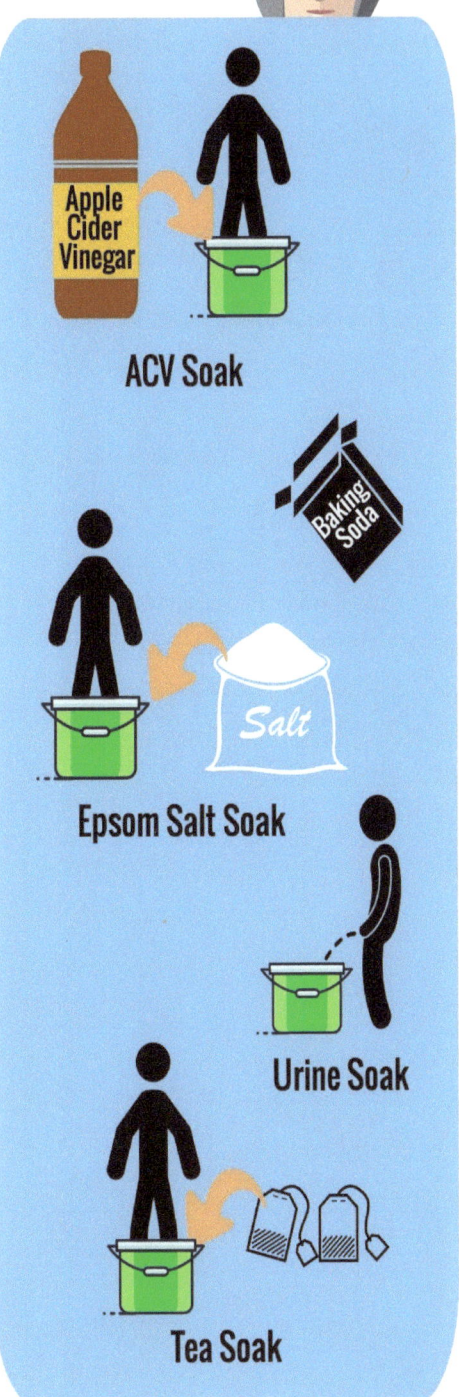

- ACV Soak
- Epsom Salt Soak
- Baking Soda
- Urine Soak
- Tea Soak

Foot Pain

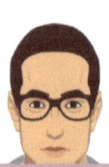
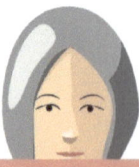

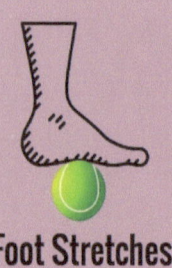
Foot Stretches

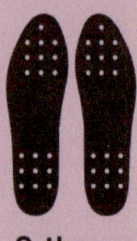
Orthoses

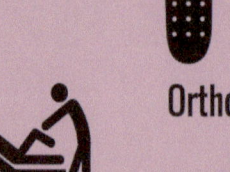
Physical Therapy

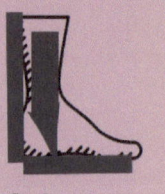
Splinting At Night

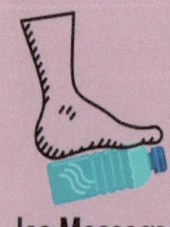
Ice Massage

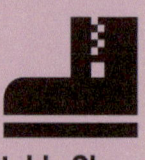
Stable Shoes

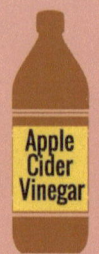

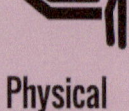
Foot Stretches

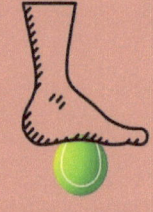
Grapefruit Seed Extract

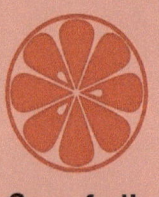
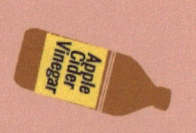
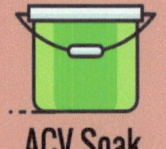
ACV Soak

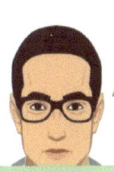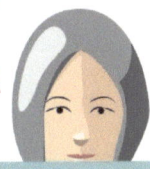

Gallstones

- Ursodiol
- Lithotripsy
- Cholecystectomy
- Ursodeoxycholic Acid

- ACV & Apple Juice
- Food Diary
- Gallstone Flush: Apple Juice, Epsom Salt, Olive Oil, Grapefruit Juice
- Exercise
- Fish Oil
- Multivitamin
- Turmeric

Gastritis

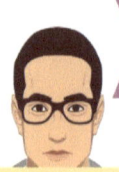
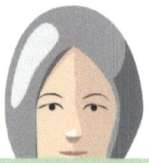

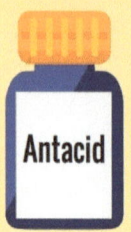
Antacid

Sucralfate

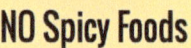
NO Spicy Foods

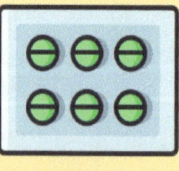
Antibiotics

Elimination Diet
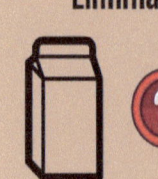  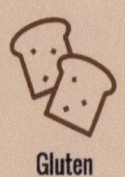
Lactose — Gluten

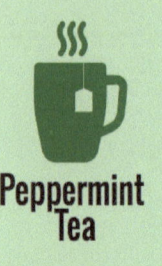
Peppermint Tea   **Ginger Tea**

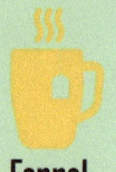
Fennel Tea

Reduce Stress

Avoid ✗
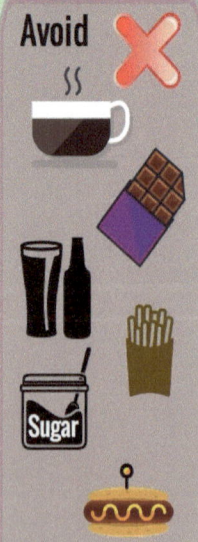

Eat ✓
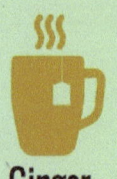
Kefir
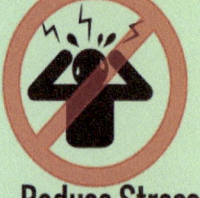
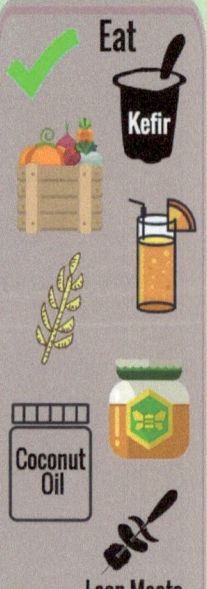
Coconut Oil
Lean Meats

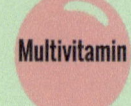
Multivitamin

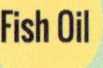
Fish Oil

Gingivitis

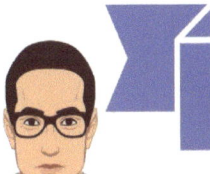
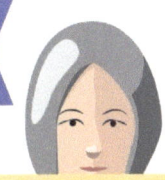

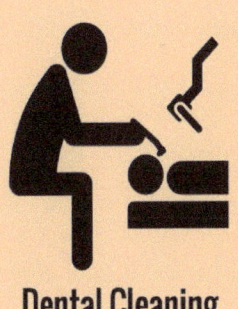
Dental Cleaning

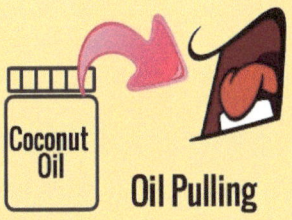
Oil Pulling

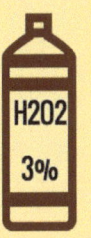
H2O2 3%

Baking Soda

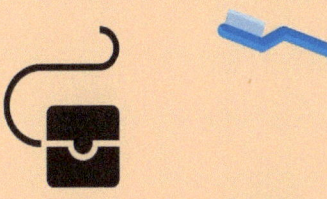

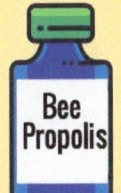
Turmeric

Mouth Rinse

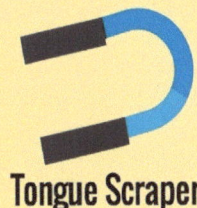
Bee Propolis / **Tongue Scraper**

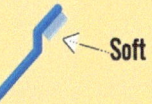
Soft
Soft Brush

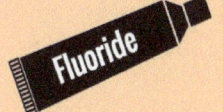

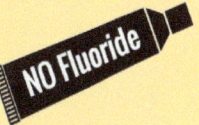
NO Fluoride

Fluoride

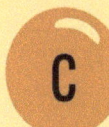
C

Fish Oil

Gout

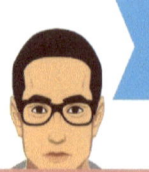
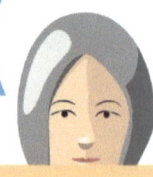

Medical Treatment
- NSAID
- Colchicine
- Corticosteroid
- Allopurinol
- Febuxostat
- Probenecid
- Less Alcohol
- More Water

Alternative Treatment
- Apple Cider Vinegar
- Baking Soda
- Cherries
- Garlic
- Multivitamin
- Fish Oil
- Chelation Therapy
- Lose Weight

Hair Loss

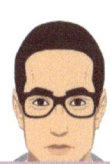
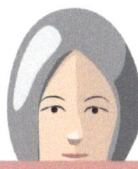
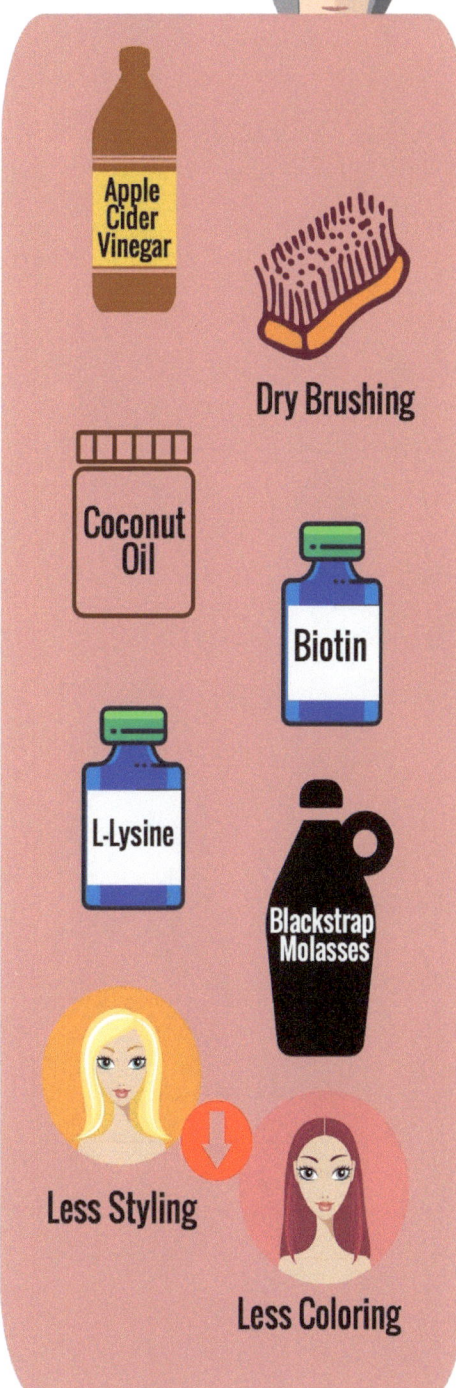

- Finasteride
- Minoxidil
- Hair Transplant
- Hair Piece
- Wig

Hangover

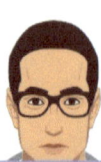
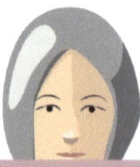
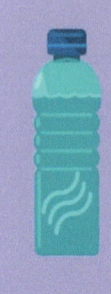
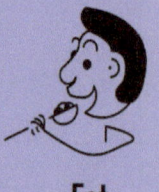

Eat

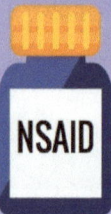

NSAID

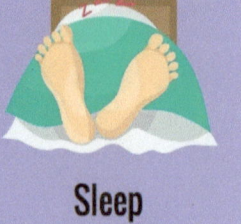

Sleep

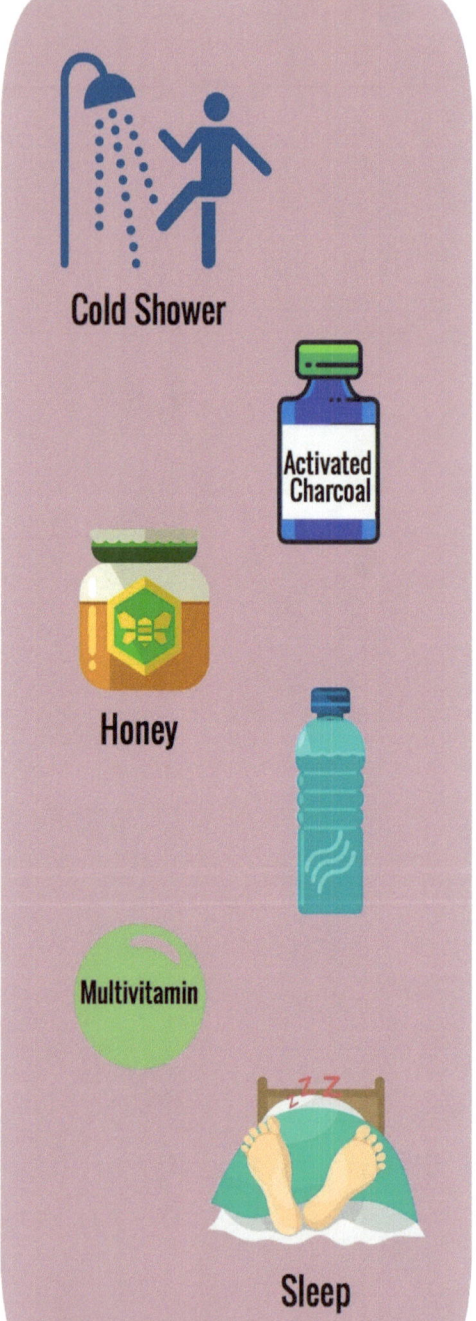

Cold Shower

Activated Charcoal

Honey

Multivitamin

Sleep

Hay Fever

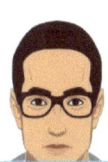
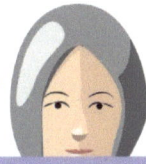

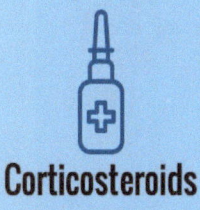
Corticosteroids

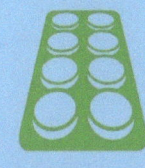
Antihistamines

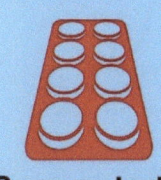
Decongestants

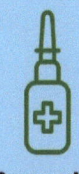
Cromolyn Sodium

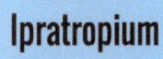
Ipratropium

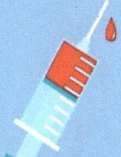
Allergy Shots

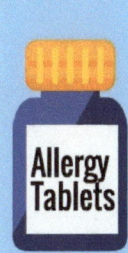
Allergy Tablets

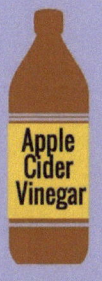
Apple Cider Vinegar

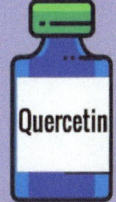
Quercetin

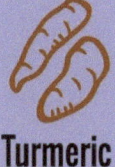
Turmeric

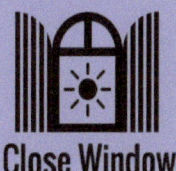
Close Window

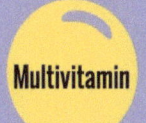
Multivitamin

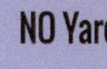
Fish Oil

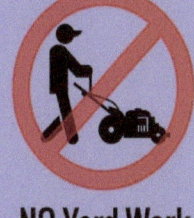
NO Yard Work

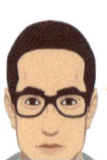 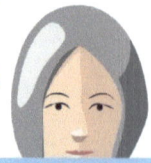

Headaches

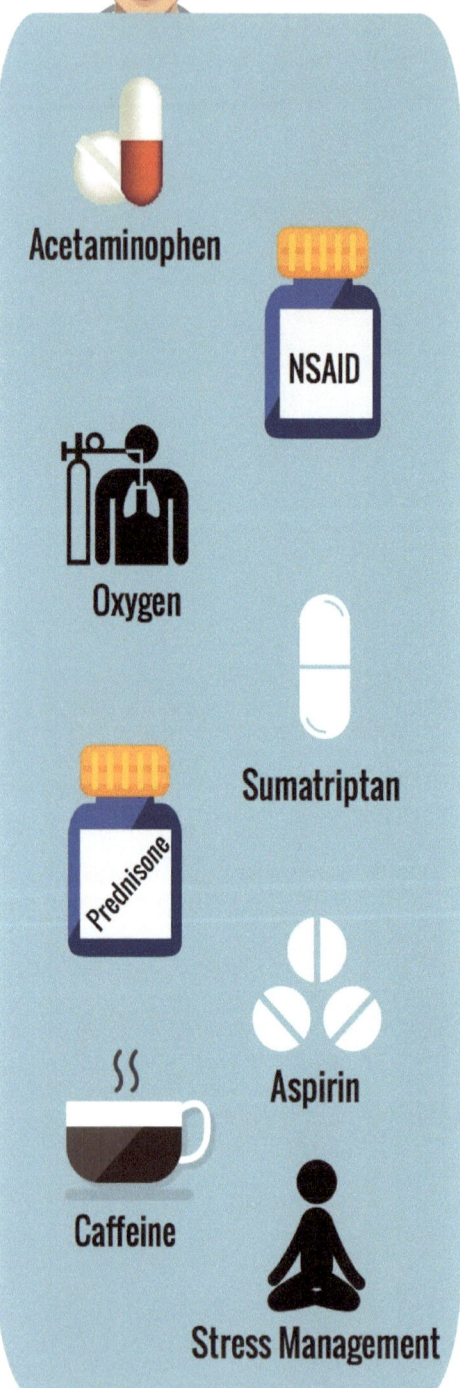
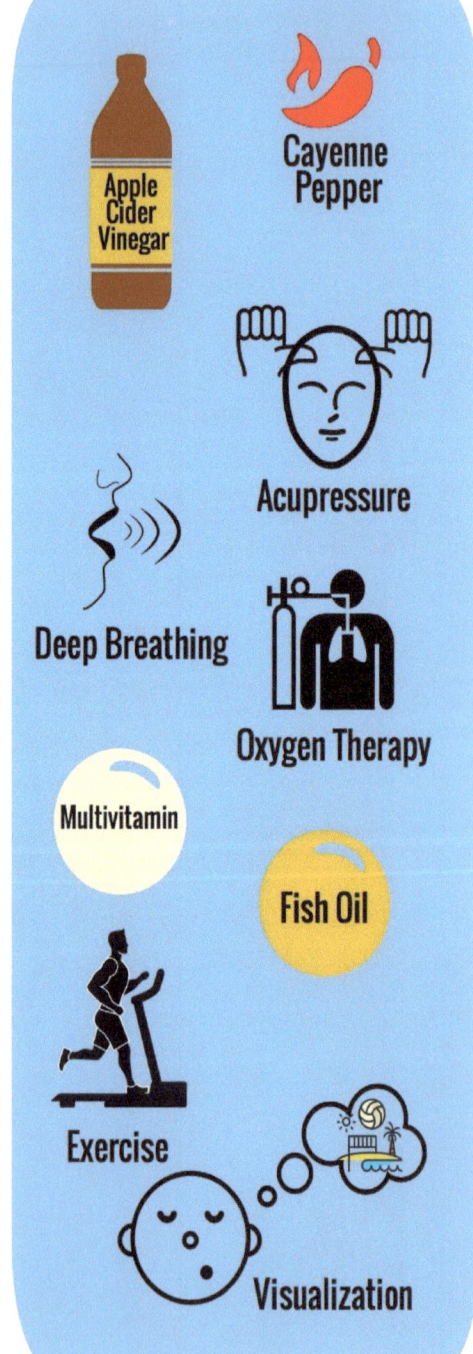

Hearing Loss

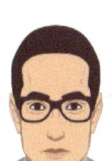
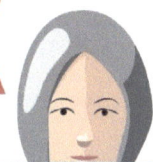

Medical Treatments

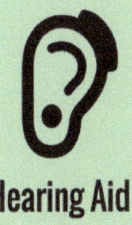
Hearing Aid

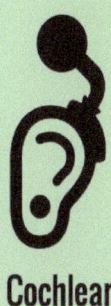
Cochlear Implant

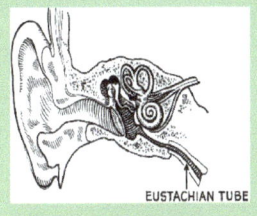
Middle Ear Implant

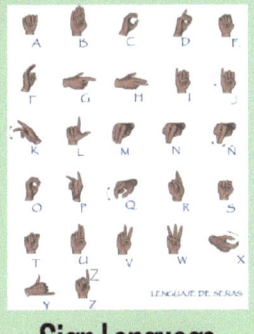
Sign Language

Natural Remedies & Prevention

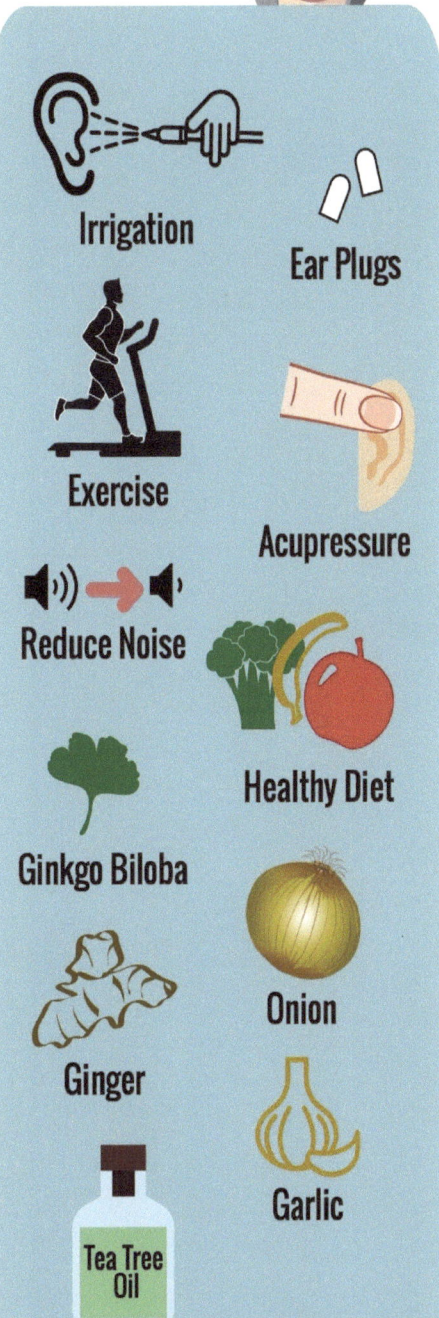

- Irrigation
- Ear Plugs
- Exercise
- Acupressure
- Reduce Noise
- Healthy Diet
- Ginkgo Biloba
- Onion
- Ginger
- Garlic
- Tea Tree Oil

Heartburn

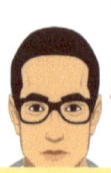
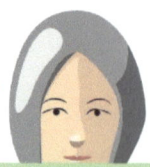
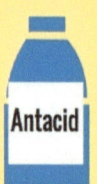
Antacid

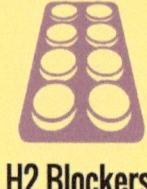
H2 Blockers

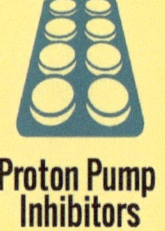
Proton Pump Inhibitors

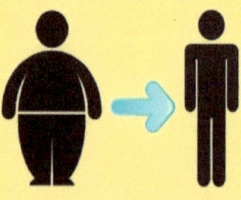
Lose Weight

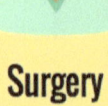
Surgery

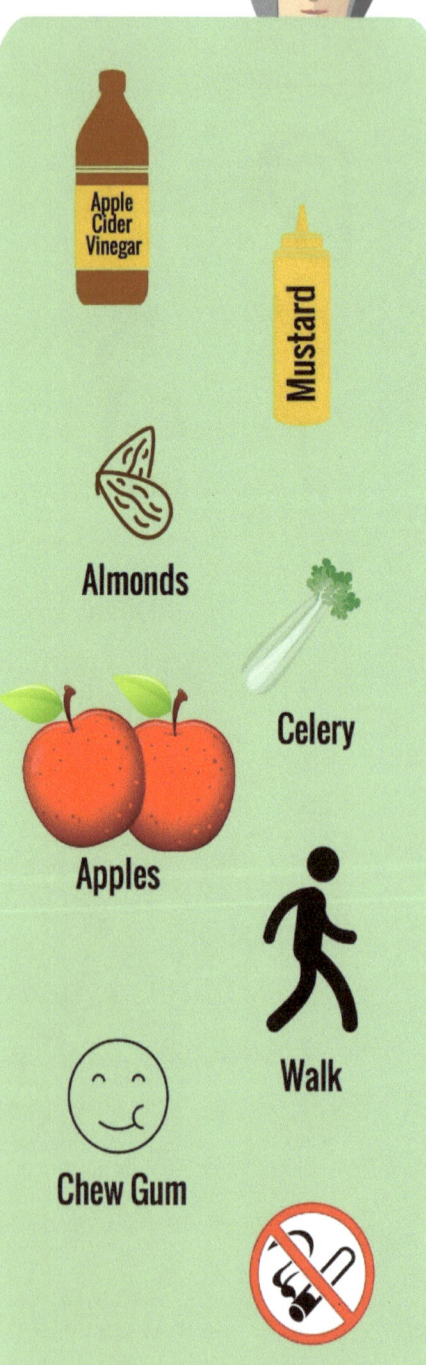
Apple Cider Vinegar
Mustard
Almonds
Celery
Apples
Walk
Chew Gum

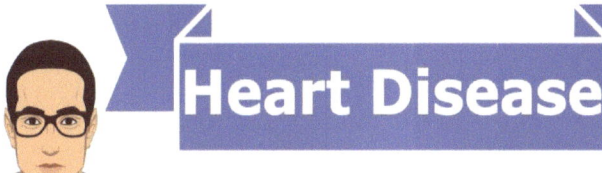
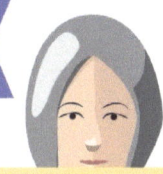

Heart Disease

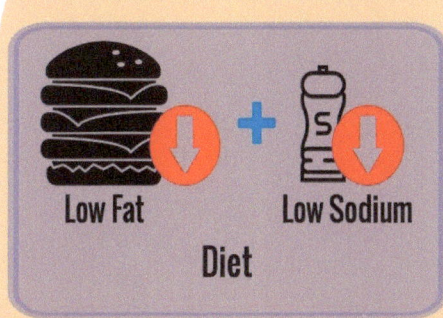

Diet
- Low Fat + Low Sodium

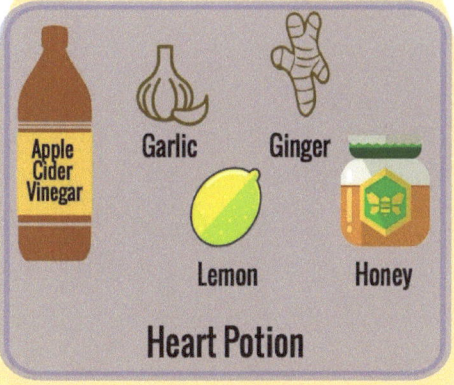

Heart Potion
- Apple Cider Vinegar
- Garlic
- Ginger
- Lemon
- Honey

 Exercise

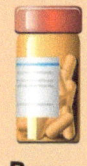 Drugs (Varies)

 Cayenne Pepper (No Smoking)

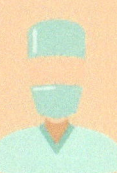 Surgery

 (No Smoking)

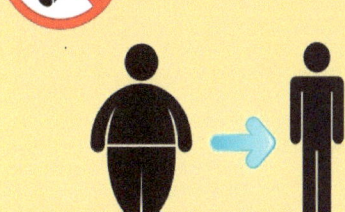 Lose Weight

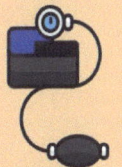 Control Blood Pressure

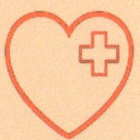 Control Cholesterol

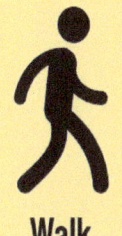 Walk

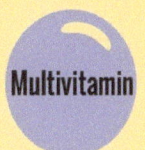 Multivitamin

 Manage Stress

Heart Palpitations

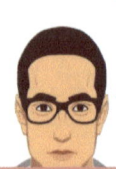
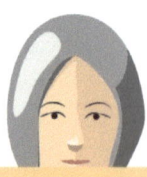
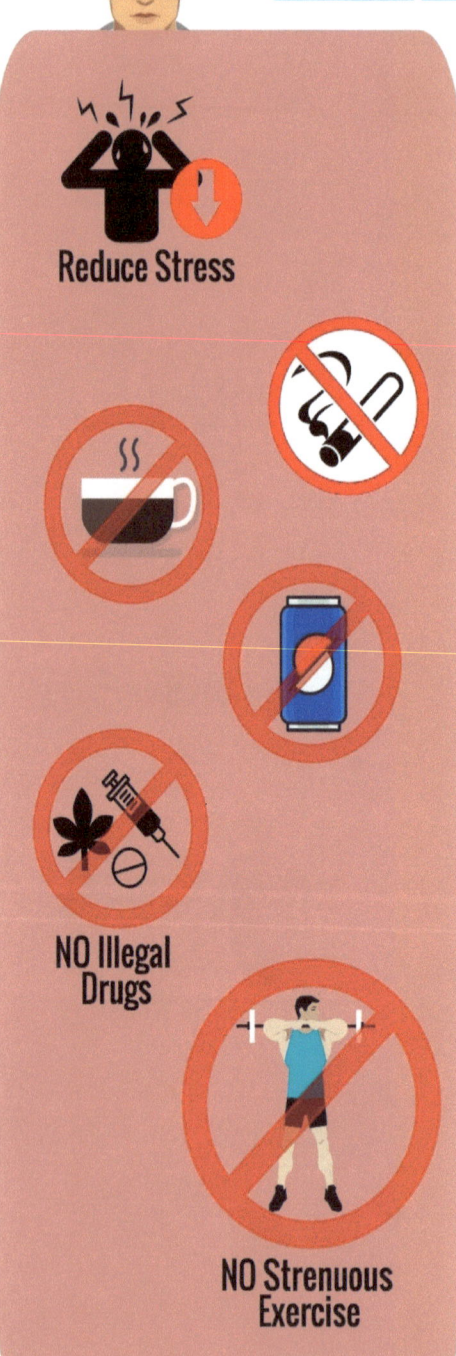
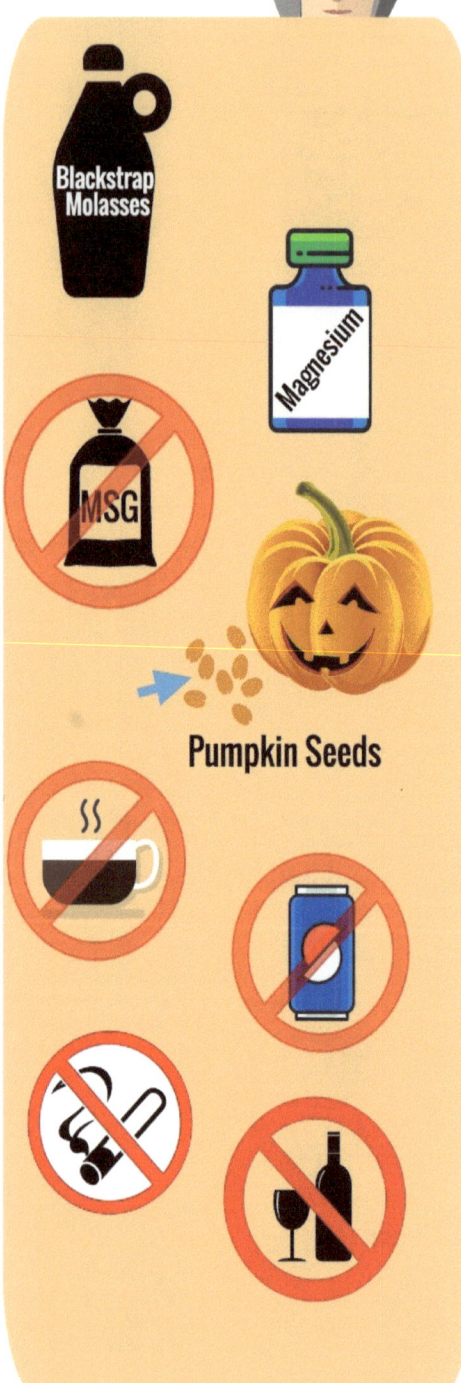

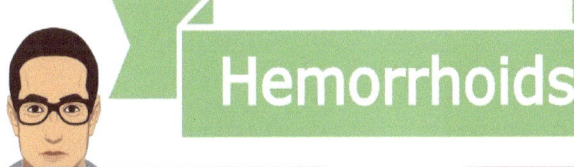

Hemorrhoids

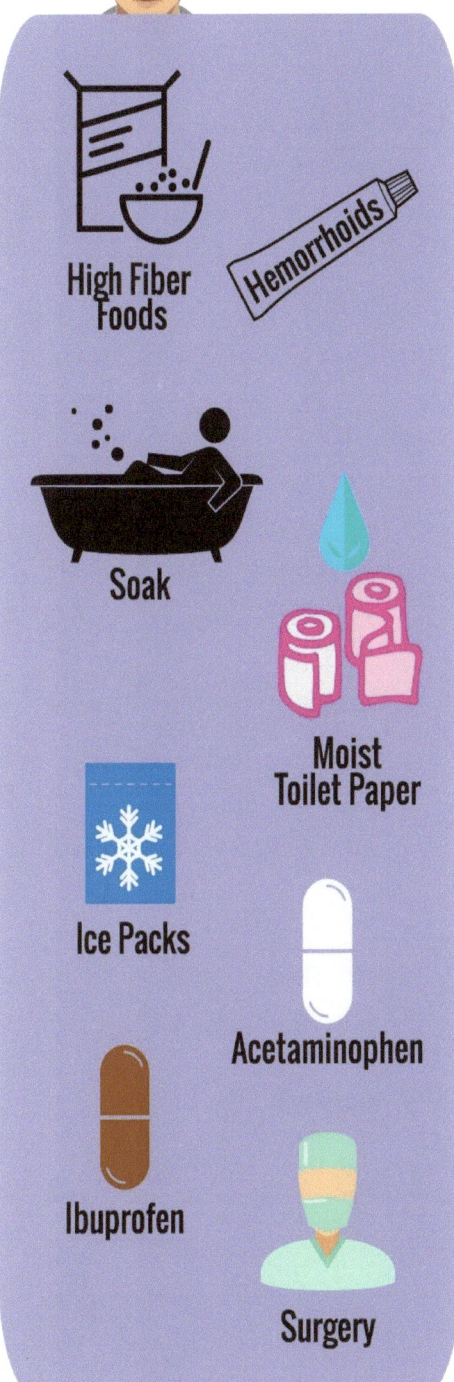

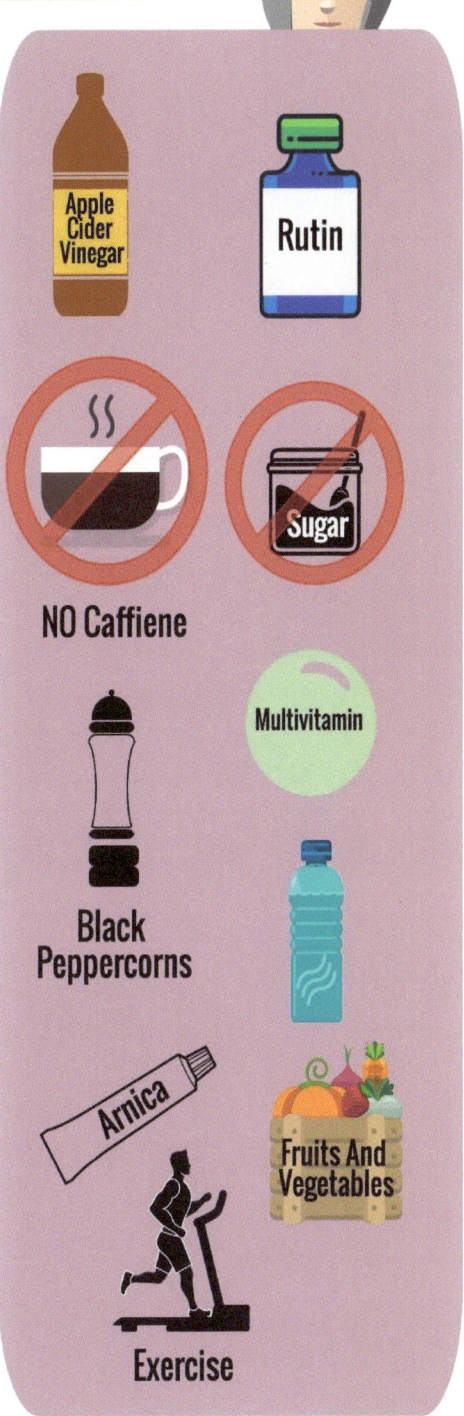

Hepatitis

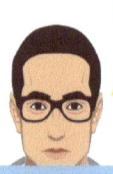
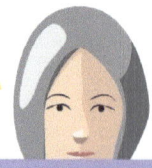

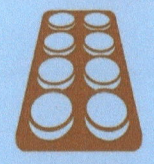 Lamivudine
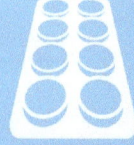 Adefovir

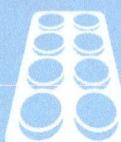 Telbivudine
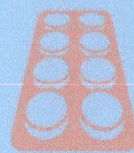 Entecavir

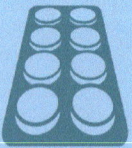 Ribavirin
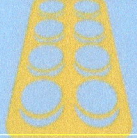 Sofosbuvir

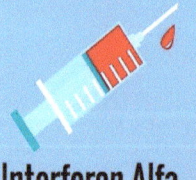 Interferon Alfa

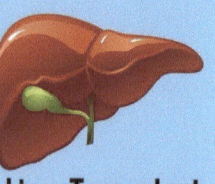 Liver Transplant

Vaccine

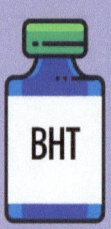 BHT

H2O2 3%

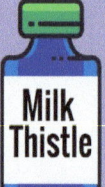 Milk Thistle

Colloidal Silver

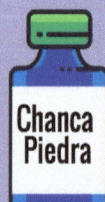 Chanca Piedra

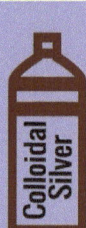
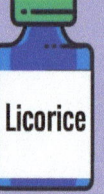 Licorice

Hiccups

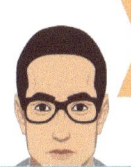
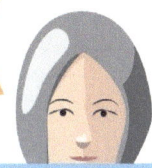

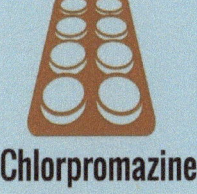
Chlorpromazine

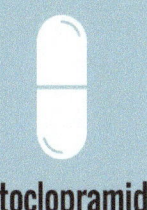
Metoclopramide

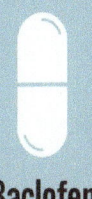
Baclofen

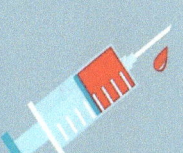
Anesthetic Injection

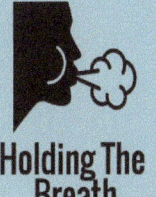
Holding The Breath

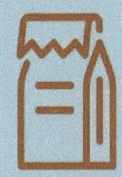
Breathe Into Paper Bag

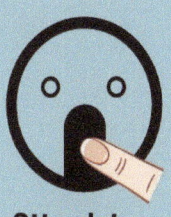
Stimulate Gagging

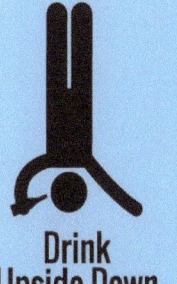
Drink Upside Down

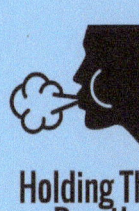
Holding The Breath

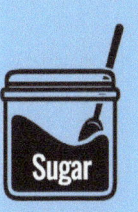
Sugar

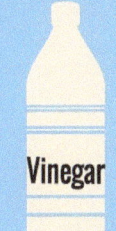
Vinegar

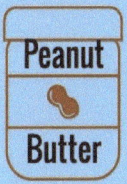
Peanut Butter

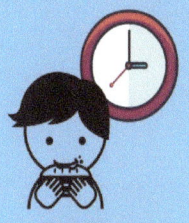
Eat Slower

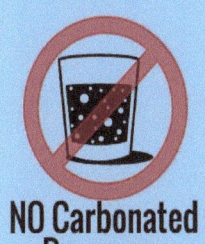
NO Carbonated Beverages

High Blood Pressure

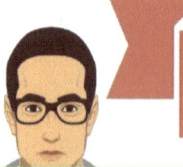
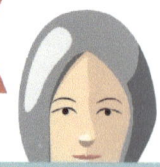
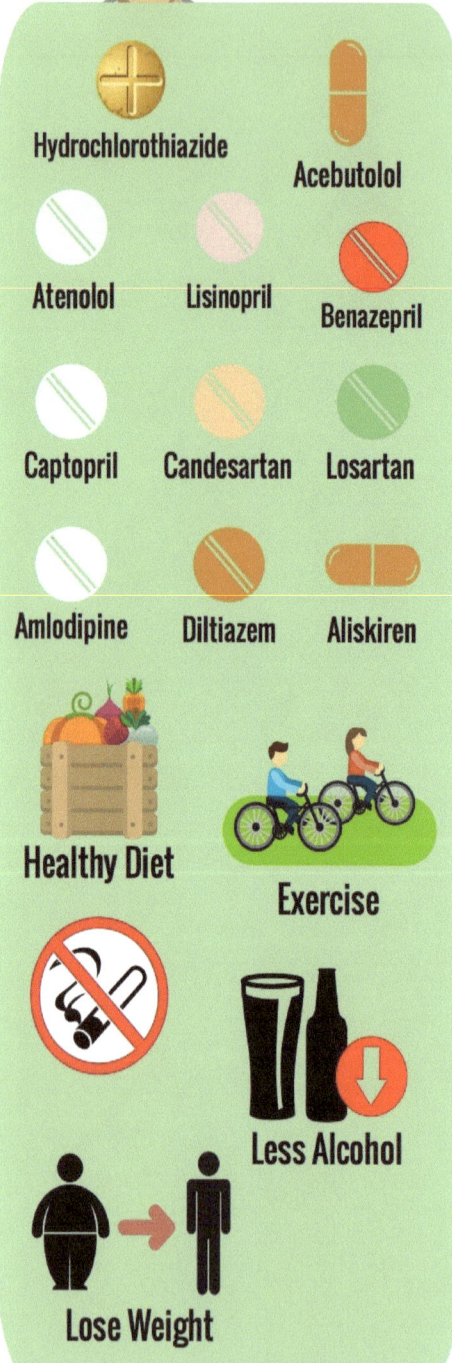
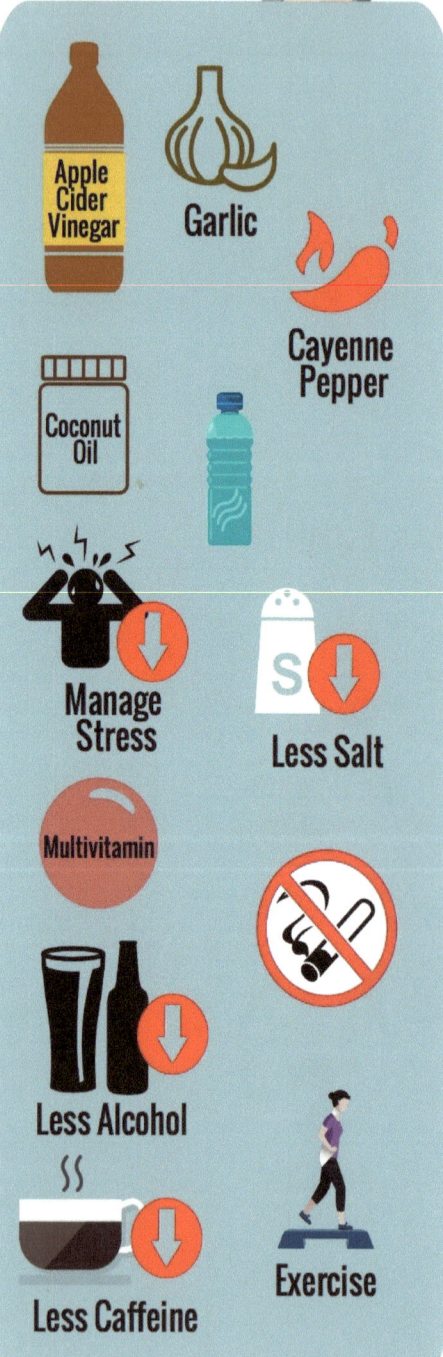

Hives

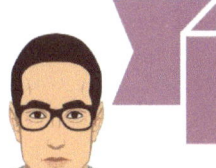
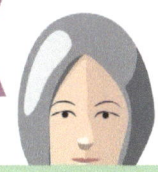

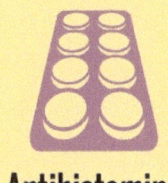
Antihistamine

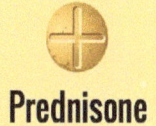
Prednisone

Avoid The Triggers

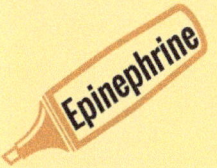
Epinephrine

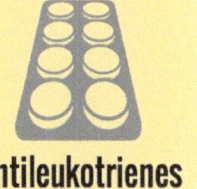
Antileukotrienes

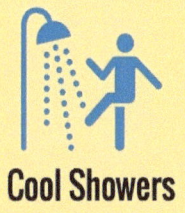
Cool Showers

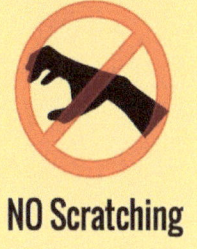
NO Scratching

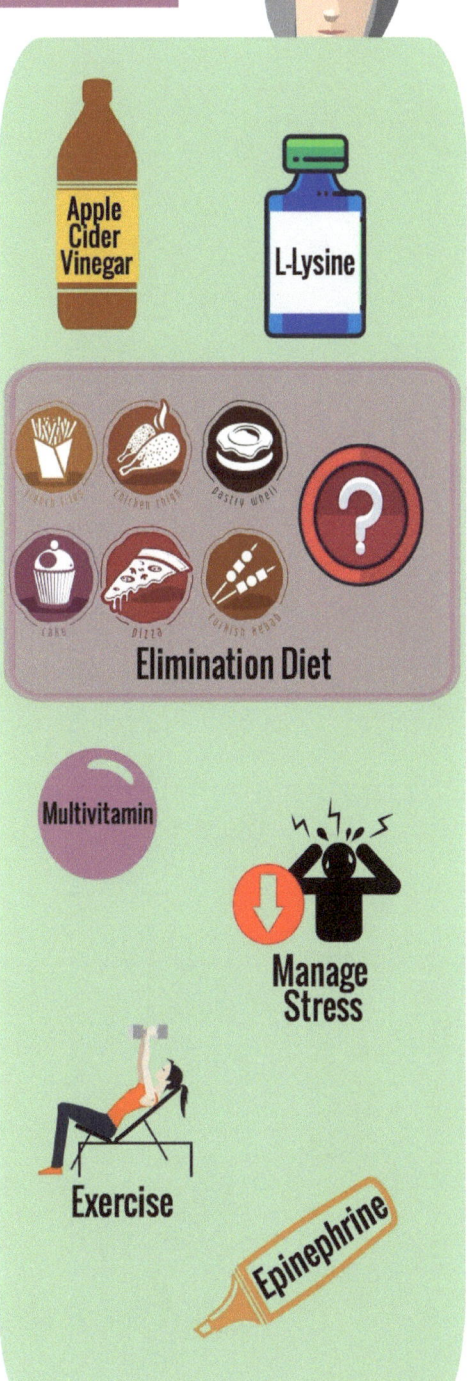

Apple Cider Vinegar • L-Lysine • Elimination Diet • Multivitamin • Manage Stress • Exercise • Epinephrine

Insomnia

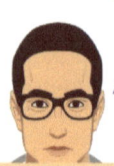
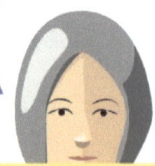

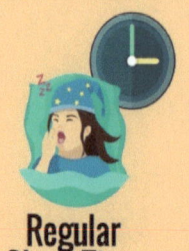
Regular Sleep Time

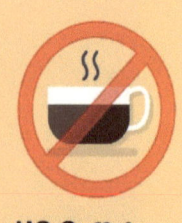
NO Caffeine After Lunch

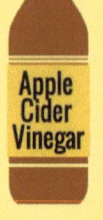
Apple Cider Vinegar

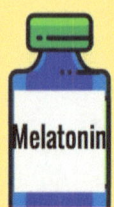
Melatonin

Reduce Stress

Flurazepam

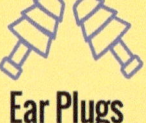
Ear Plugs

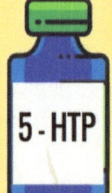
5 - HTP

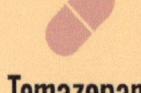
Temazepam

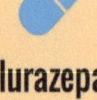
Triazolam

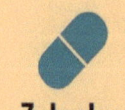
Zaleplon

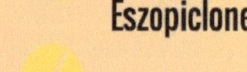
Zolpidem **Eszopiclone** **Ramelteon**

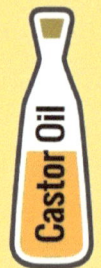
Castor Oil

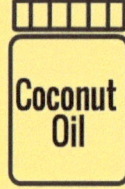
Coconut Oil

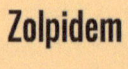
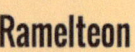

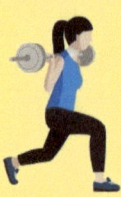
Exercise

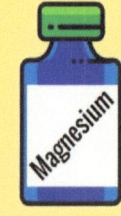
Magnesium

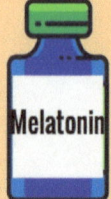
Melatonin

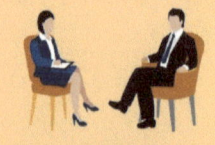
Cognitive Behavioral Therapy

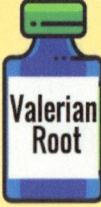
Valerian Root

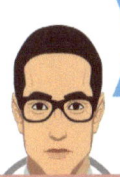 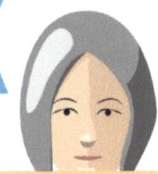

Irritable Bowel Syndrome

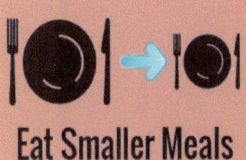
Eat Smaller Meals

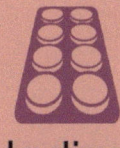
Laxatives

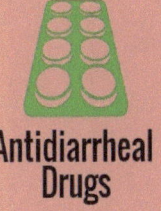
Antidiarrheal Drugs

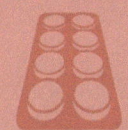
Anticholinergic Drugs

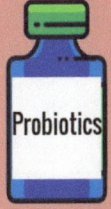
Probiotics

Hypnosis

Antidepressants

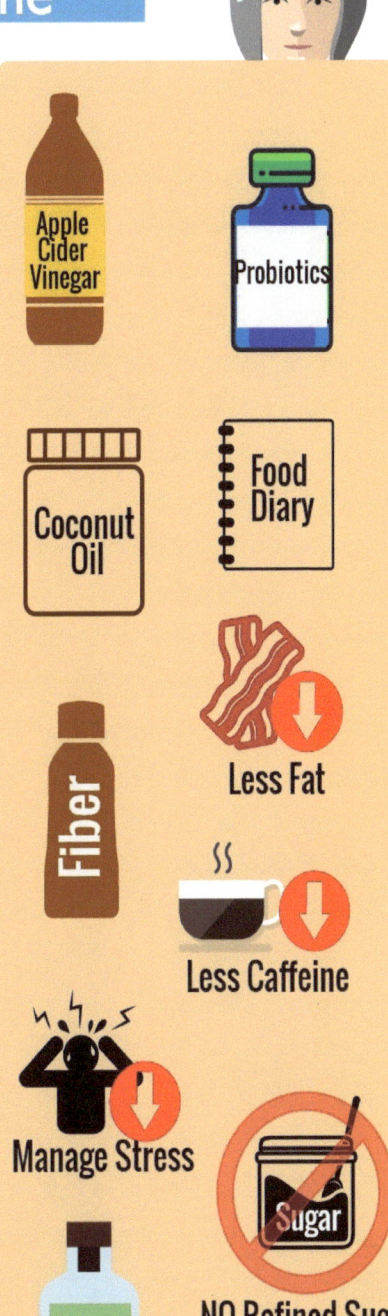

Apple Cider Vinegar

Probiotics

Coconut Oil

Food Diary

Fiber

Less Fat

Less Caffeine

Manage Stress

Peppermint Oil

NO Refined Sugar

Jock Itch

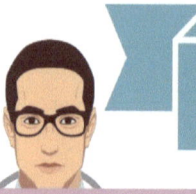
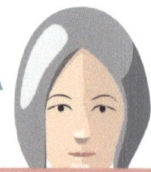

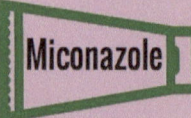
Miconazole

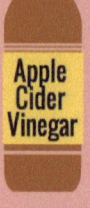
Apple Cider Vinegar

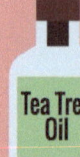
Tea Tree Oil

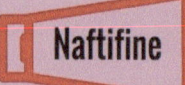
Naftifine

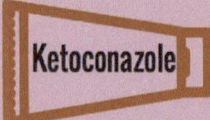
Ketoconazole

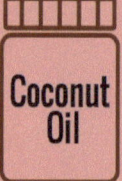
Coconut Oil

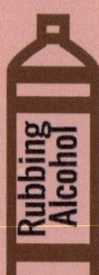
Rubbing Alcohol

Clotrimazole

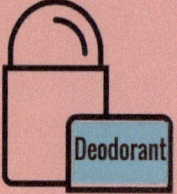
Deodorant

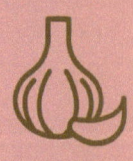
Garlic

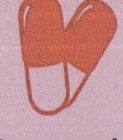
Itraconazole

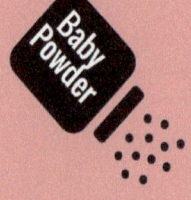
Baby Powder

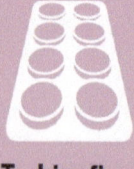
Terbinafine

Blow Dryer (On Cool)

Kidney Stones

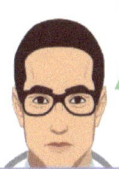
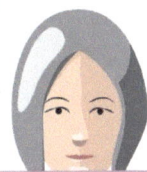

Medical Treatments

- NSAID
- Opioids
- Fluids
- Surgery
- Shockwave Lithotripsy
- Potassium Citrate

Natural Remedies

- Apple Cider Vinegar
- Lemon Juice & Olive Oil
- Chanca Piedra
- Magnesium
- Lemon Juice & Water
- B6
- Cranberry

Knee Pain

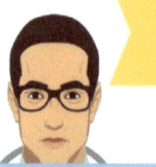
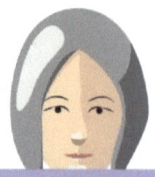
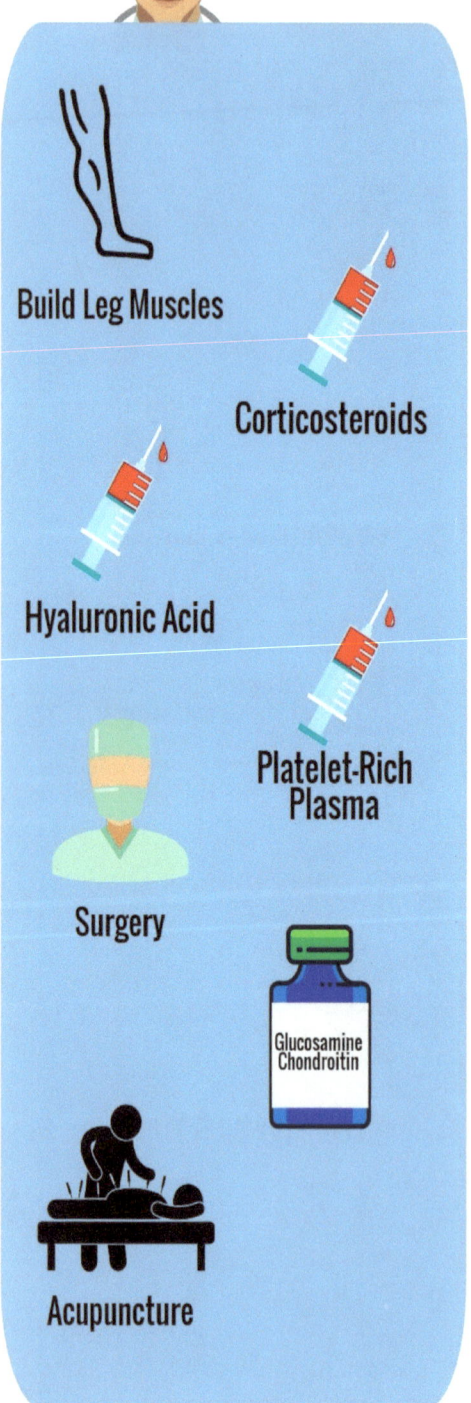
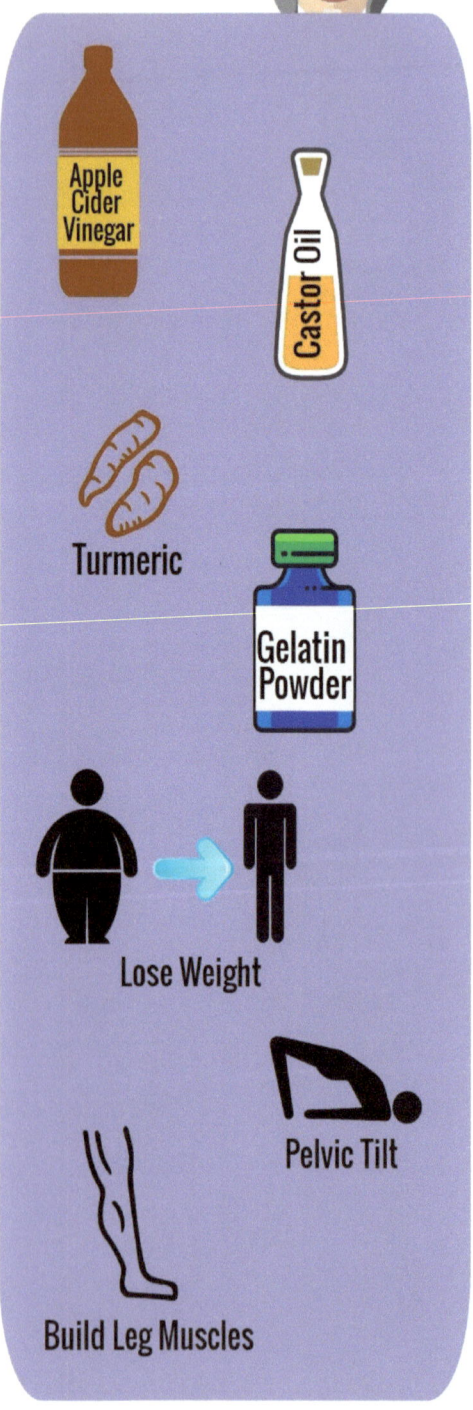

Laryngitis

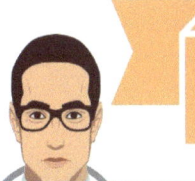
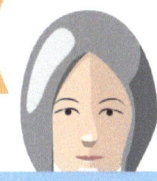
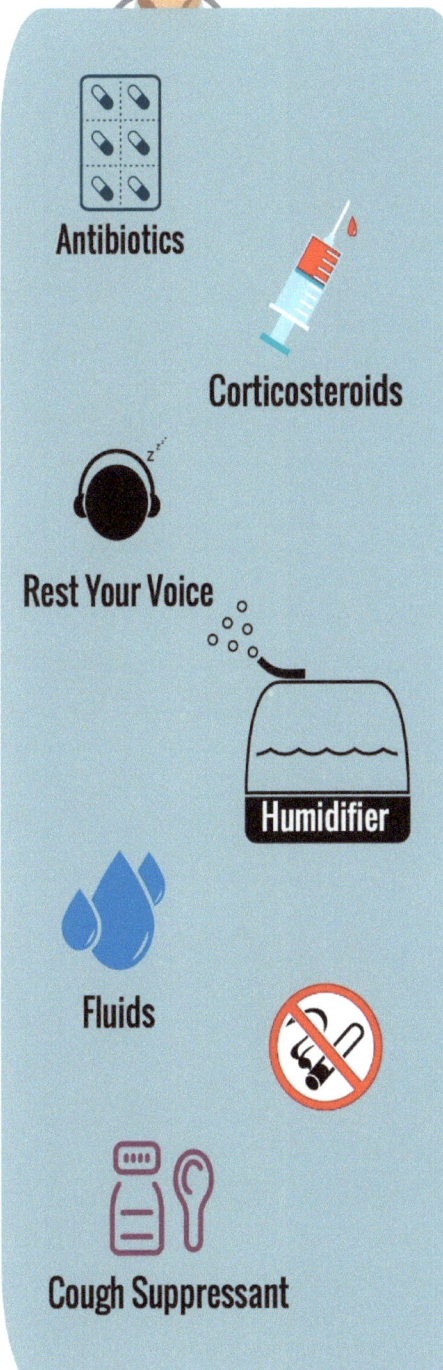
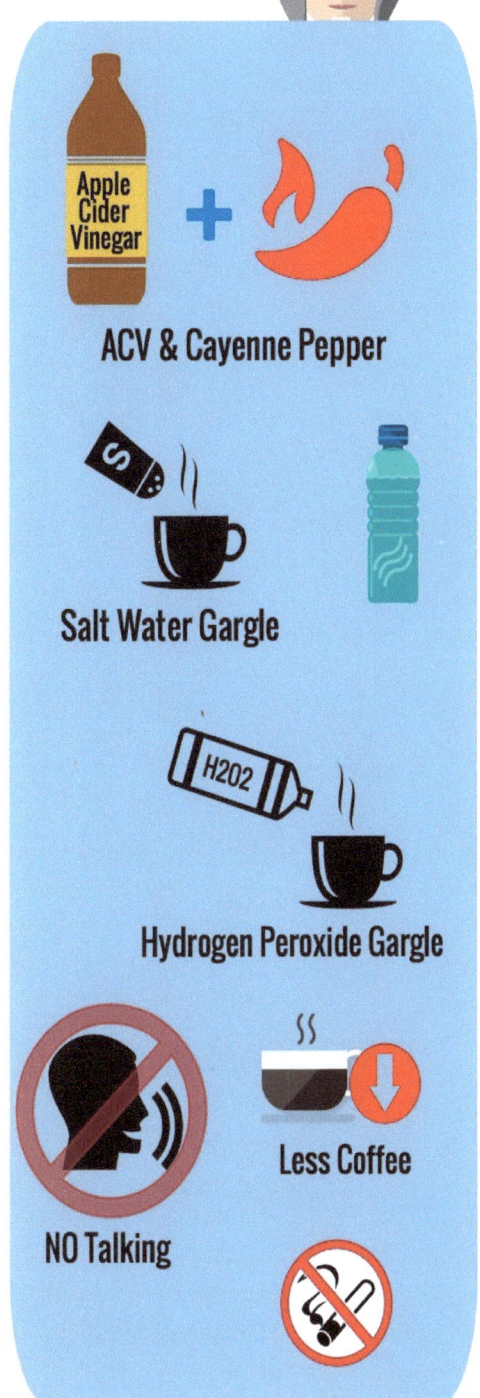

Low Blood Pressure

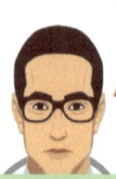
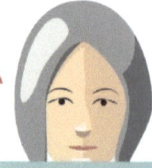

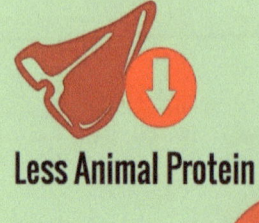
Less Animal Protein

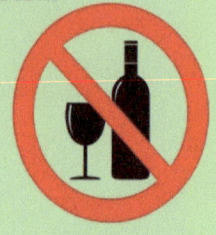

More Salt

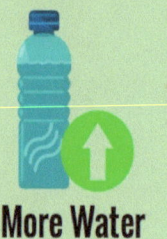
More Water

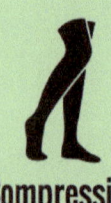
Compression Stockings

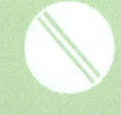
Fludrocortisone

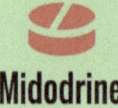
Midodrine

Low Carb Meals

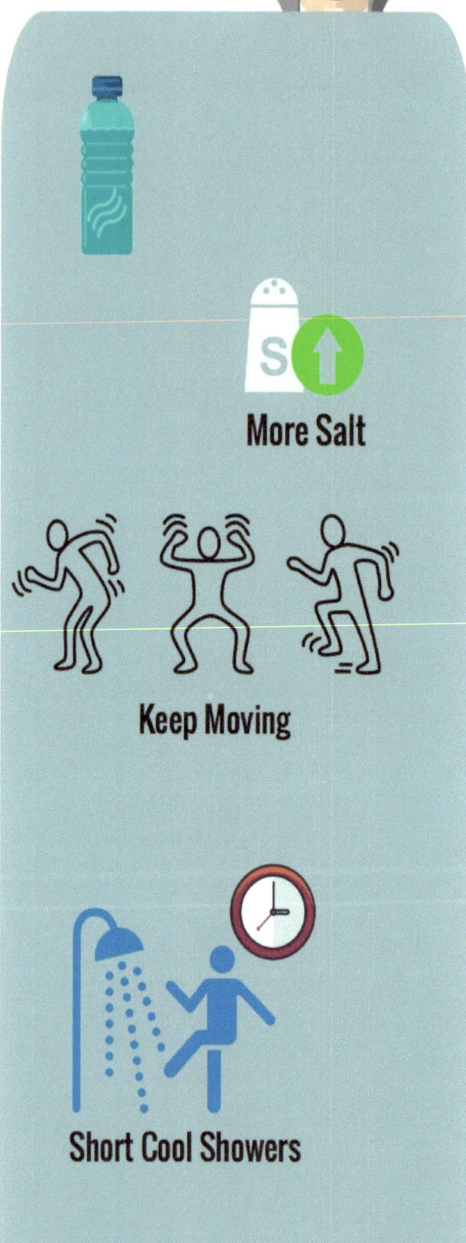

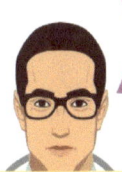 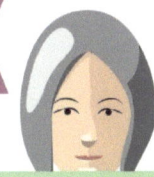

Lung Cancer

- Surgery
- Chemotherapy
- Radiation Therapy
- Afatinib
- Bevacizumab
- Ceritinib
- Crizotinib
- Palliative Care

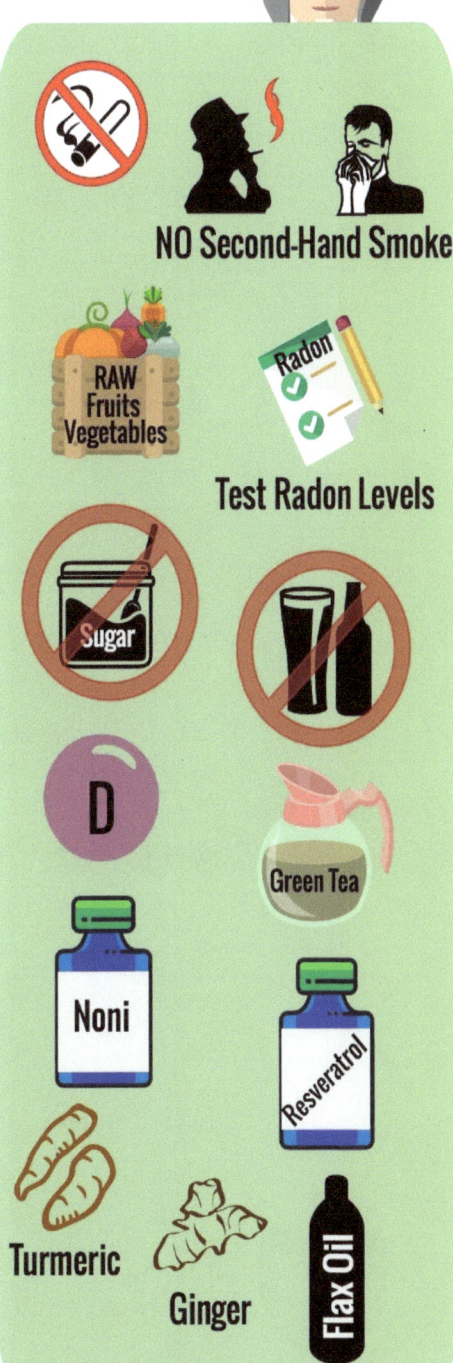

- NO Second-Hand Smoke
- RAW Fruits Vegetables
- Test Radon Levels
- No Sugar
- No Alcohol
- Vitamin D
- Green Tea
- Noni
- Resveratrol
- Turmeric
- Ginger
- Flax Oil

Lupus

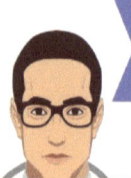
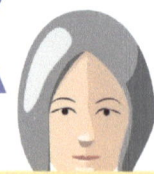

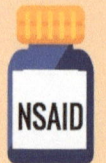 NSAID   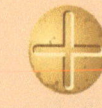 Hydroxychloroquine

 Anti-Inflammatory Diet   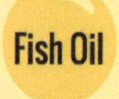 Fish Oil

Corticosteroid   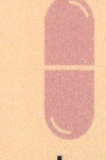 Azathioprine

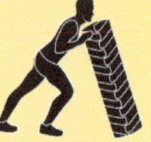 Exercise

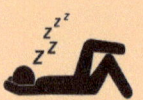 Leflunomide   Mycophenolate

 Reduce Stress   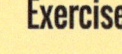 Rest

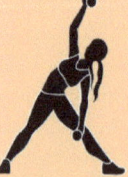 Rest   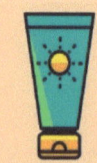 Methotrexate

 Protect From Sun   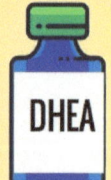 DHEA

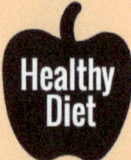 Exercise   Sunscreen

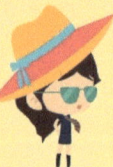 D3

 Healthy Diet

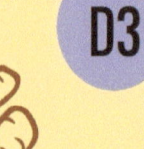 Turmeric   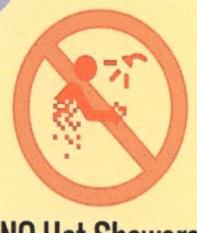 NO Hot Showers

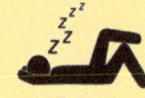

Lyme Disease

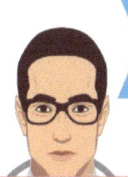
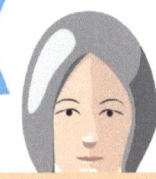
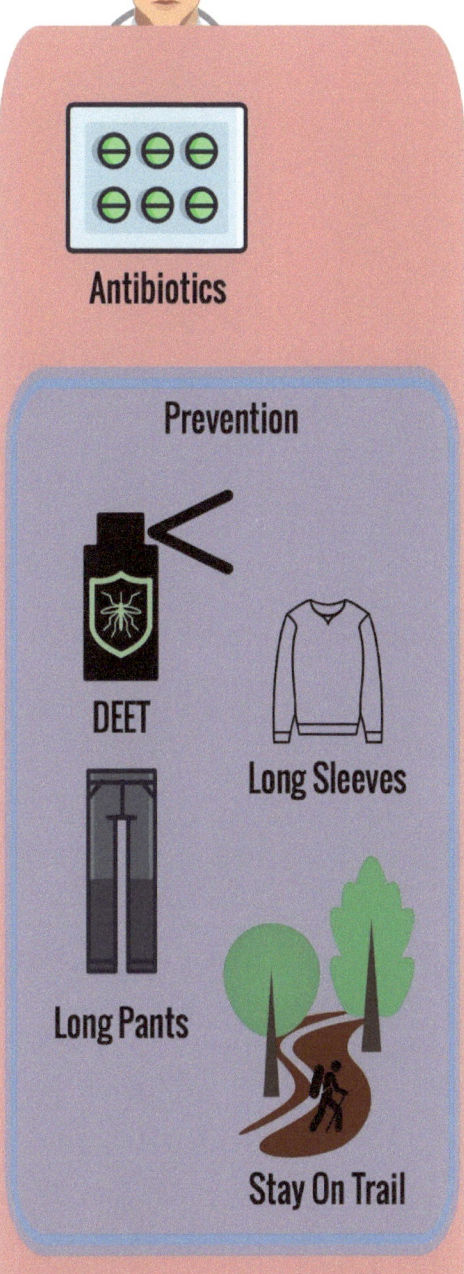
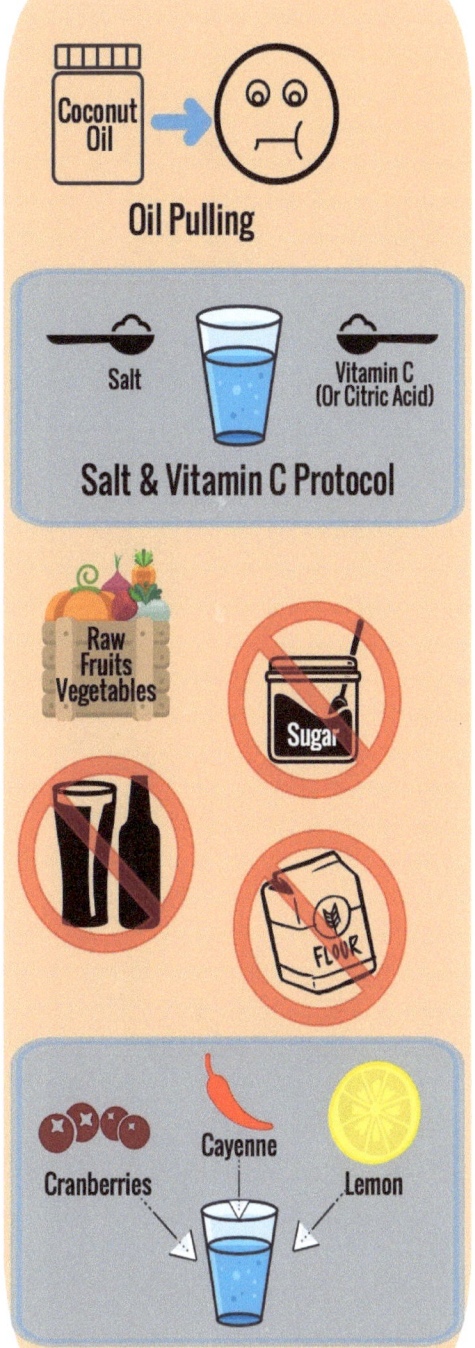

Menopause
Hormone Replacement Therapy
Estrogen
SSRI
Gabapentin
Lubricant
Sleep
Relaxation Techniques
Exercise
Apple Cider Vinegar
Soy
Trigger Diary
Less Coffee
Multivitamin
Less Chocolate
Fish Oil
Flaxseed
Sage Tea
Evening Primrose Oil
Healthy Diet
Exercise

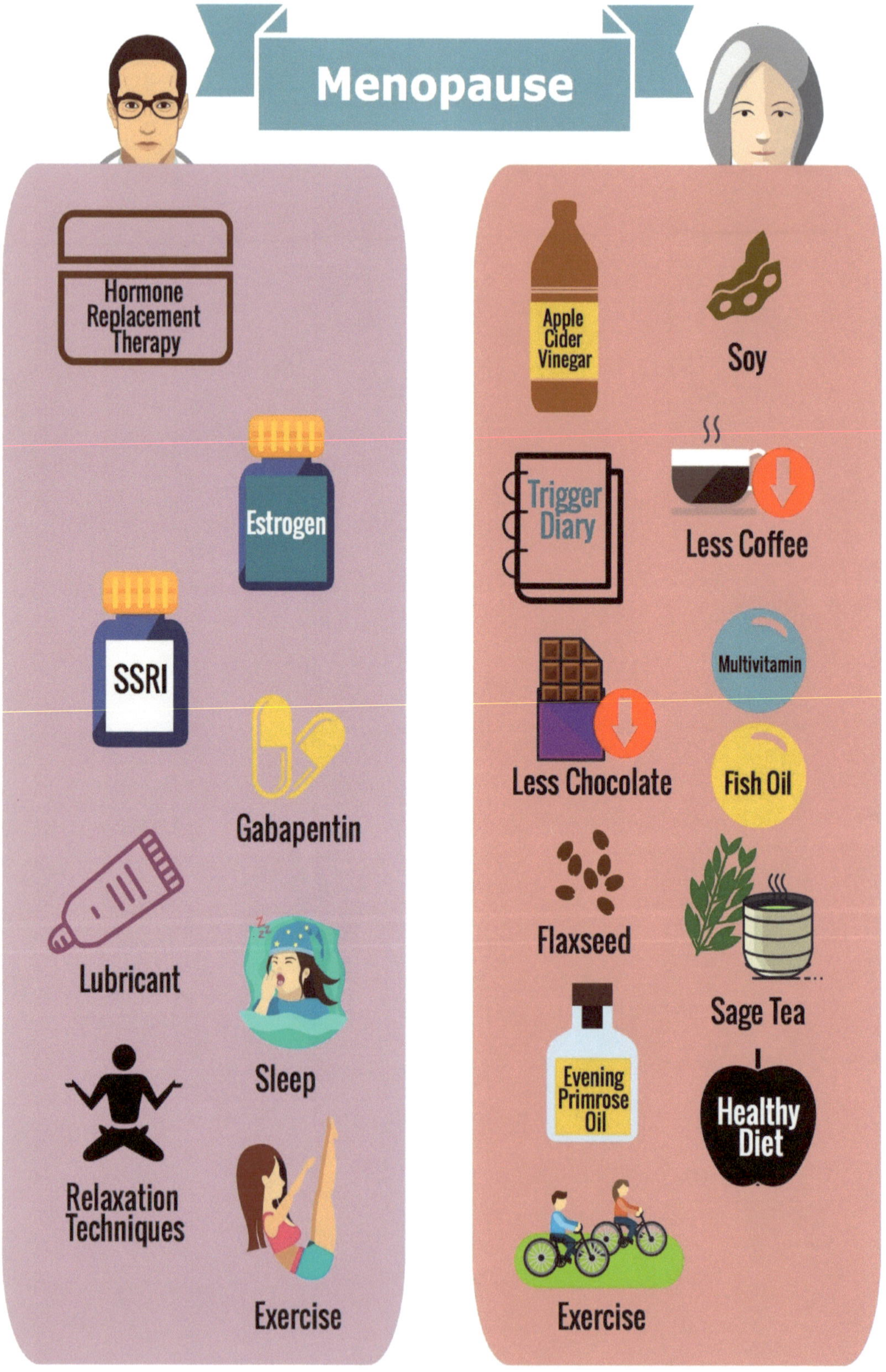

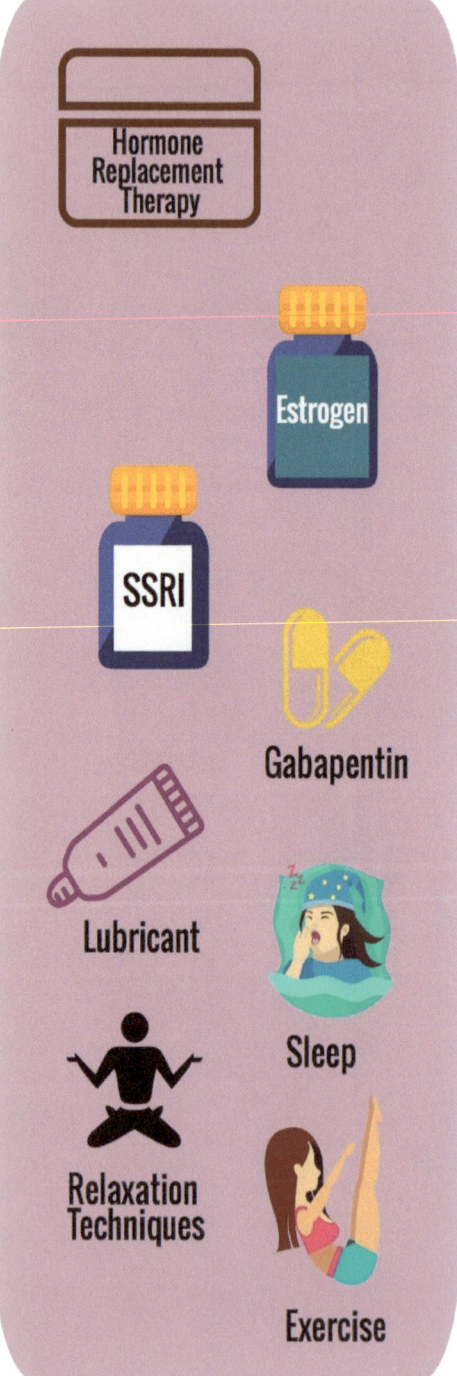

Menstrual Cramps

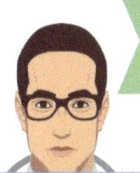
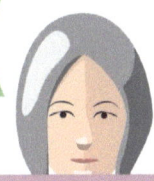
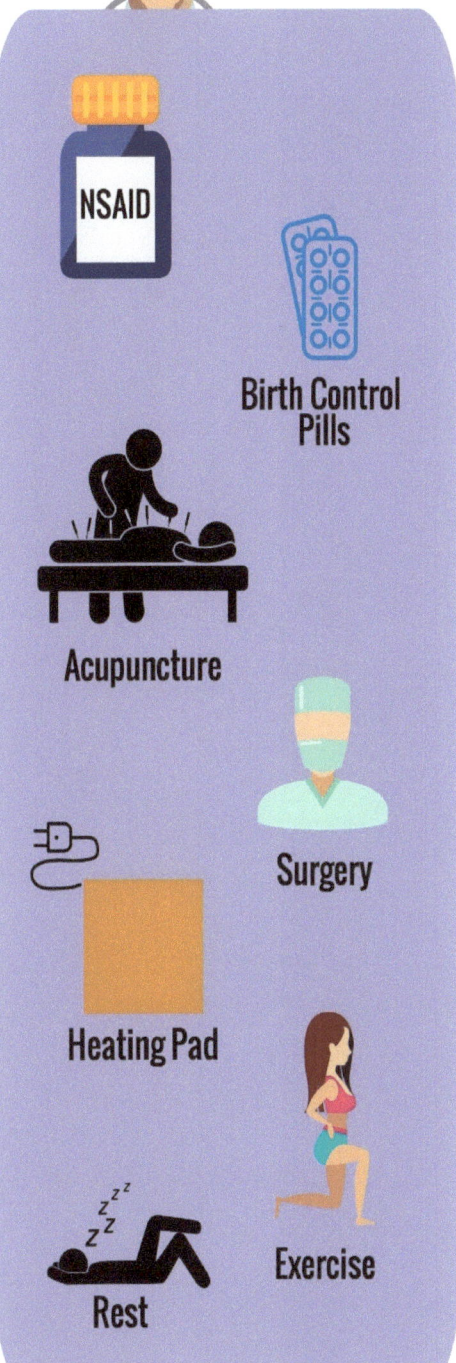
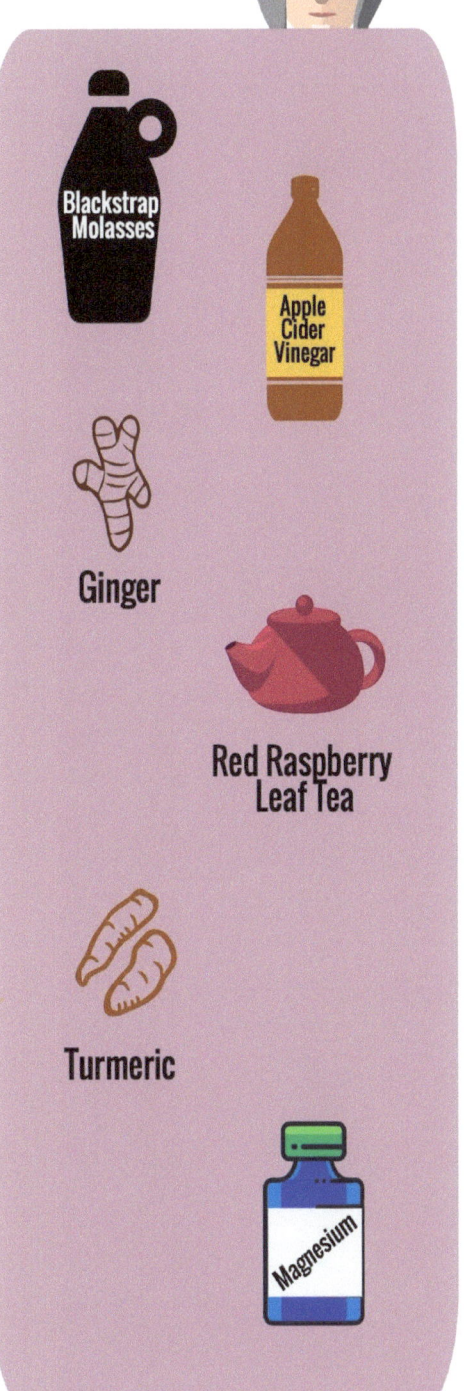

Mononucleosis

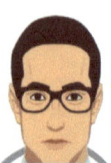
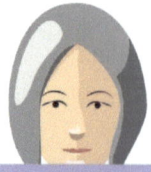

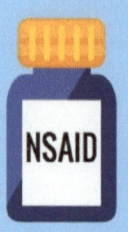 NSAID

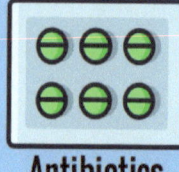 Antibiotics

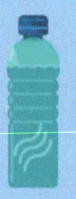

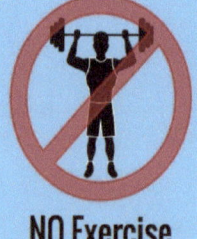 NO Exercise

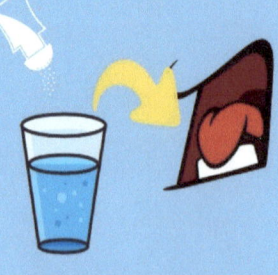 Salt Water Gargle

Coconut Oil

NO Kissing

NO Heavy Lifting

C

Cranberry Juice

Garlic

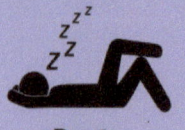
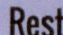
Rest

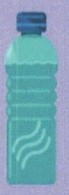

Motion Sickness

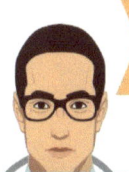
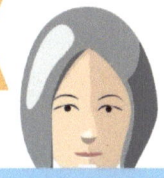
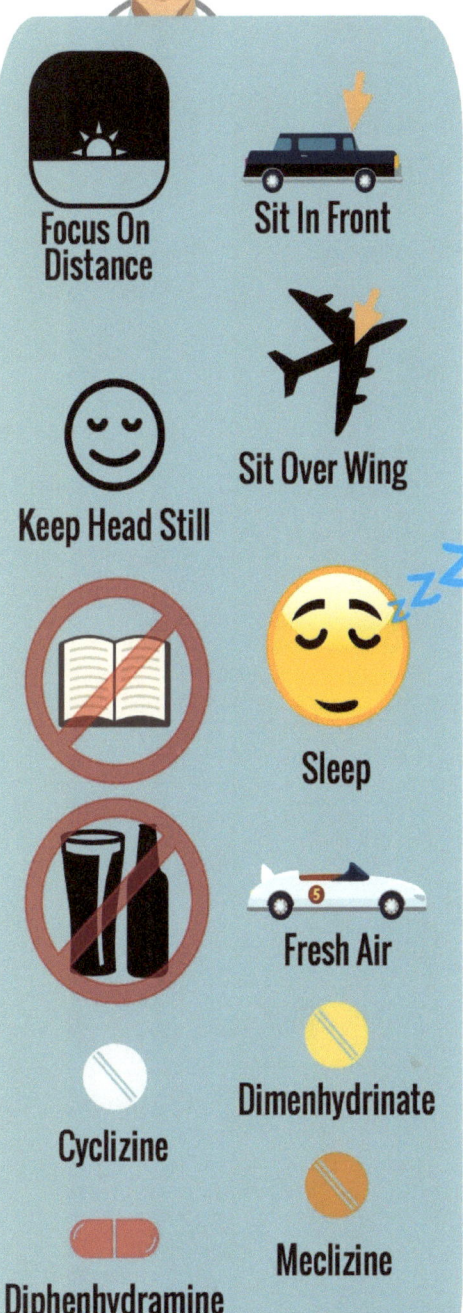

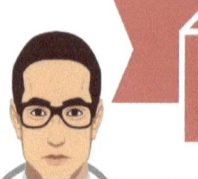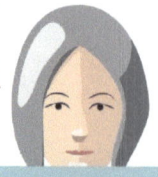

Multiple Sclerosis

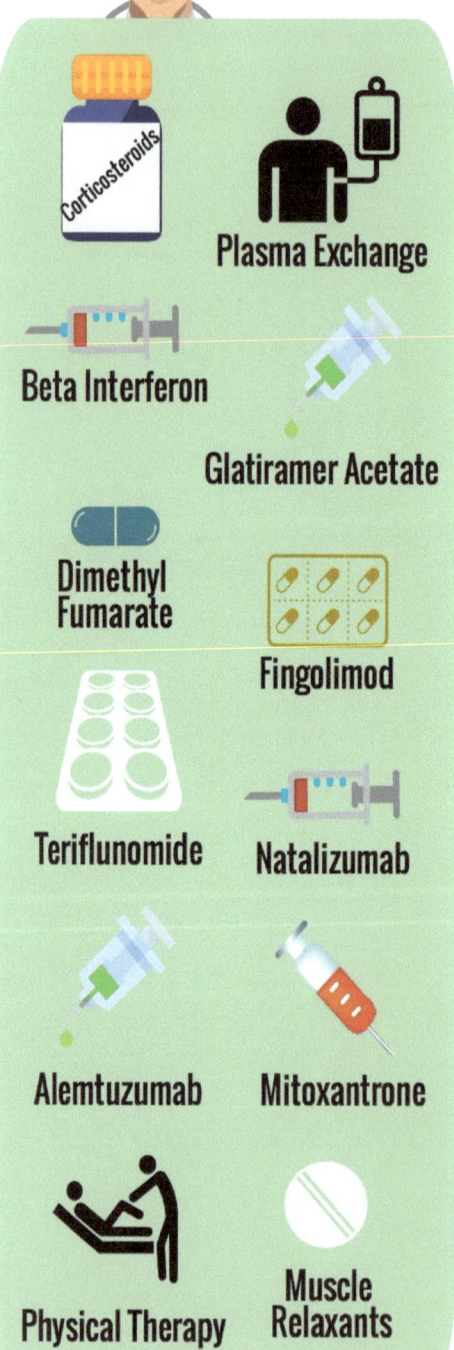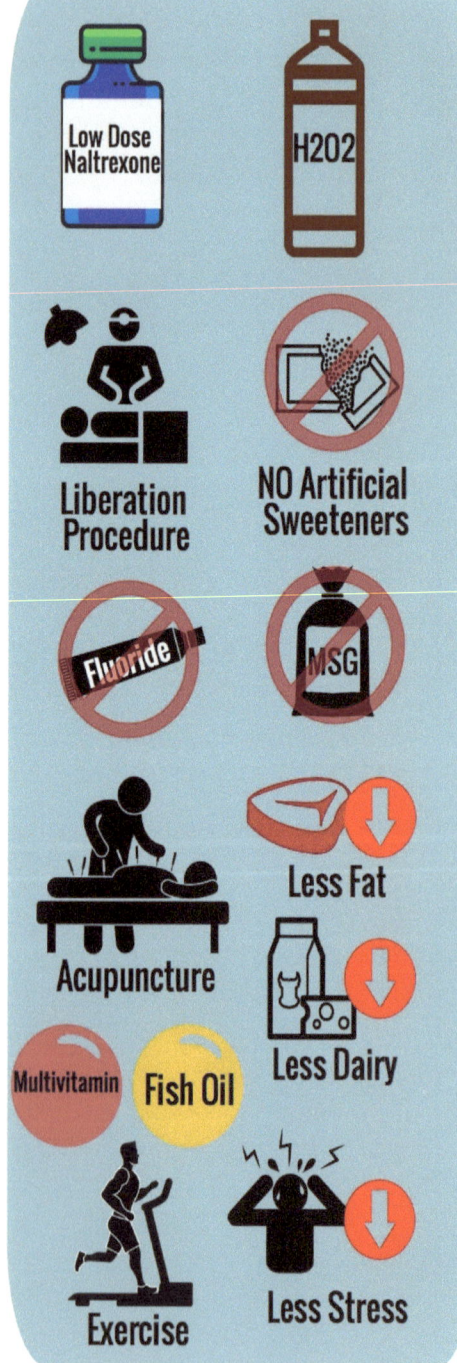

Muscle Cramps

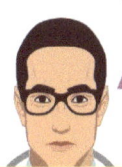
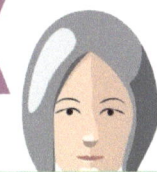

Conventional

- **Magnesium**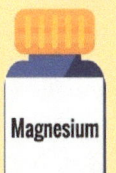
- **Potassium**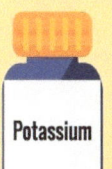
- **Stretching**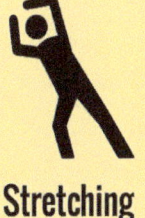
- **Fluids**
- **NO Caffeine**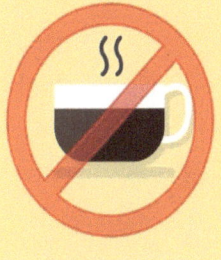

Alternative

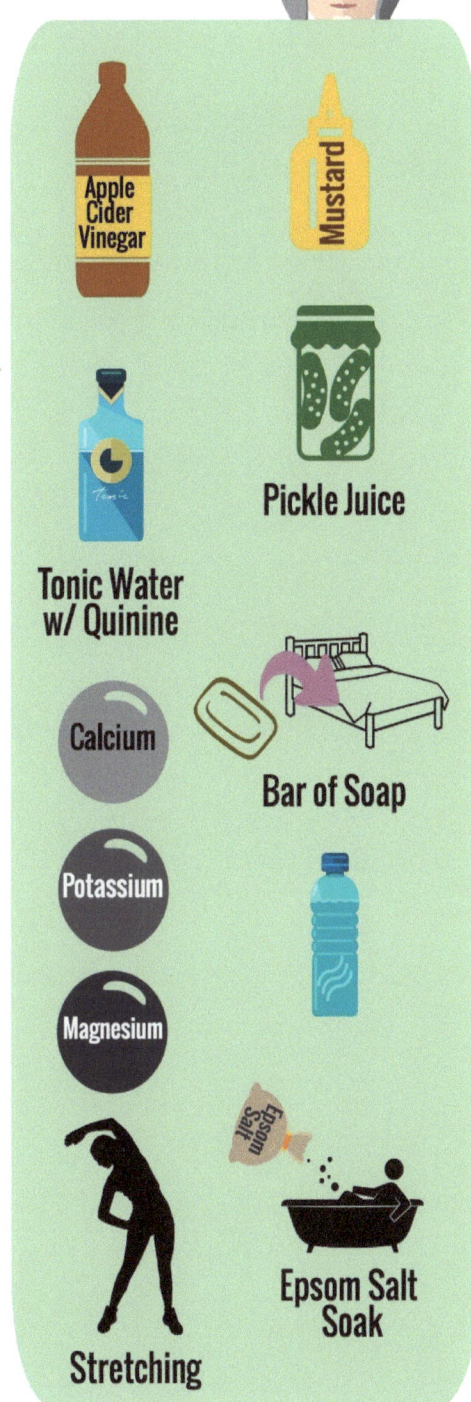

- Apple Cider Vinegar
- Mustard
- Tonic Water w/ Quinine
- Pickle Juice
- Calcium
- Bar of Soap
- Potassium
- Magnesium
- Stretching
- Epsom Salt Soak

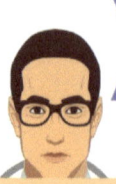 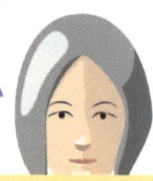

Nails

Nail Disorders

 **Brown Strip** — Melanoma

White Lines — Malnutrition

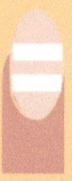 **Vertical Lines** — Age

Concave — Iron Deficiency

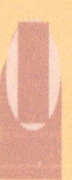 **Brittle** — Environmental Factors

Half Moon — Liver Disease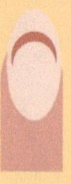

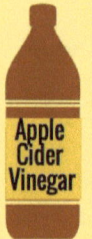 Apple Cider Vinegar

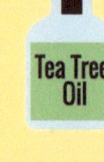 Baking Soda

 H2O2

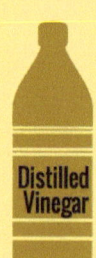 Tea Tree Oil

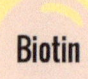 Biotin

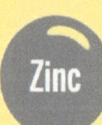 Zinc

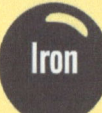 Iron

Distilled Vinegar

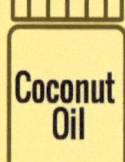 Coconut Oil

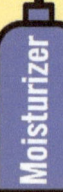 Moisturizer

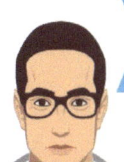 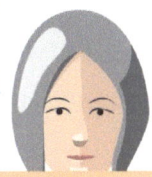

Neck & Shoulder Pain

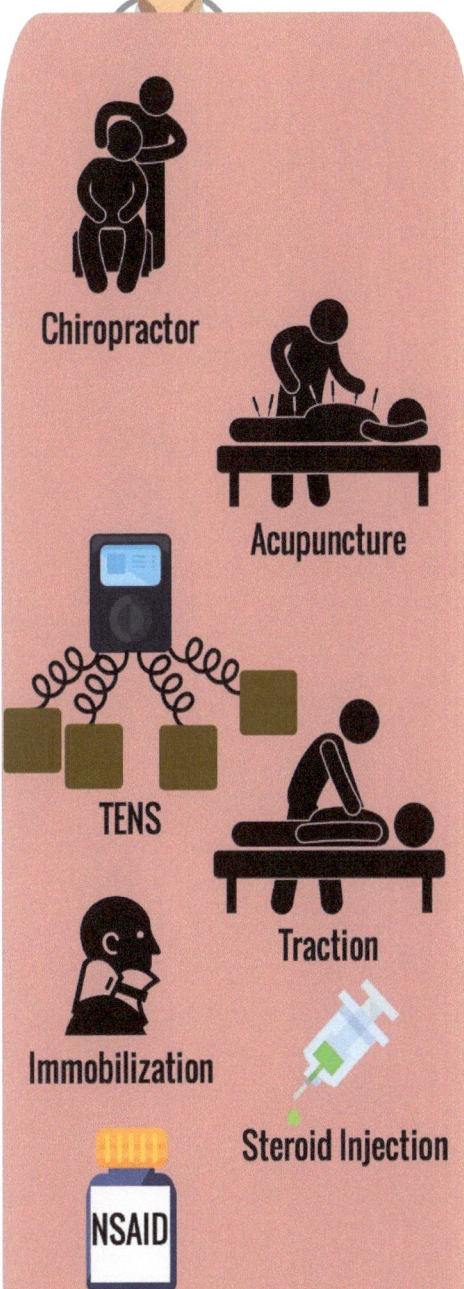

- Chiropractor
- Acupuncture
- TENS
- Traction
- Immobilization
- Steroid Injection
- NSAID

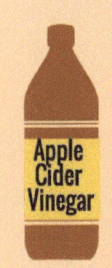 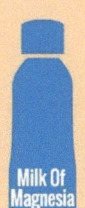

Apple Cider Vinegar · Milk Of Magnesia

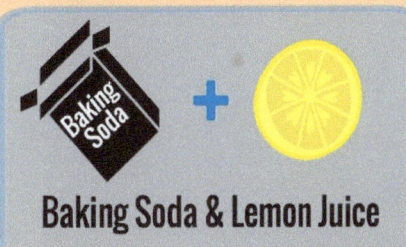

Baking Soda & Lemon Juice

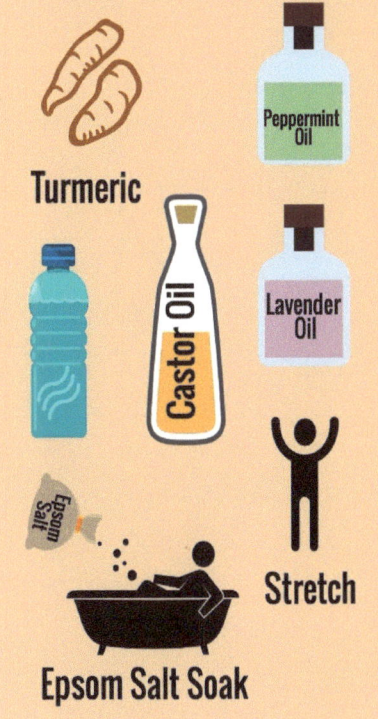

- Turmeric
- Peppermint Oil
- Castor Oil
- Lavender Oil
- Epsom Salt Soak
- Stretch

Nightmares

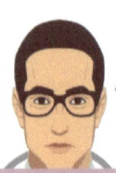
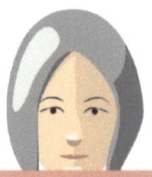
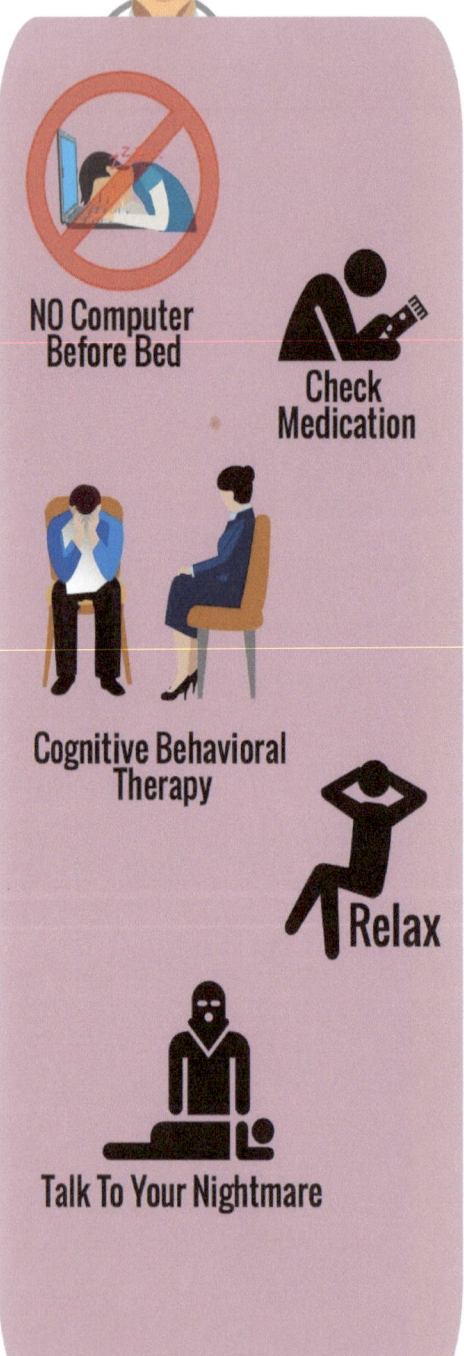
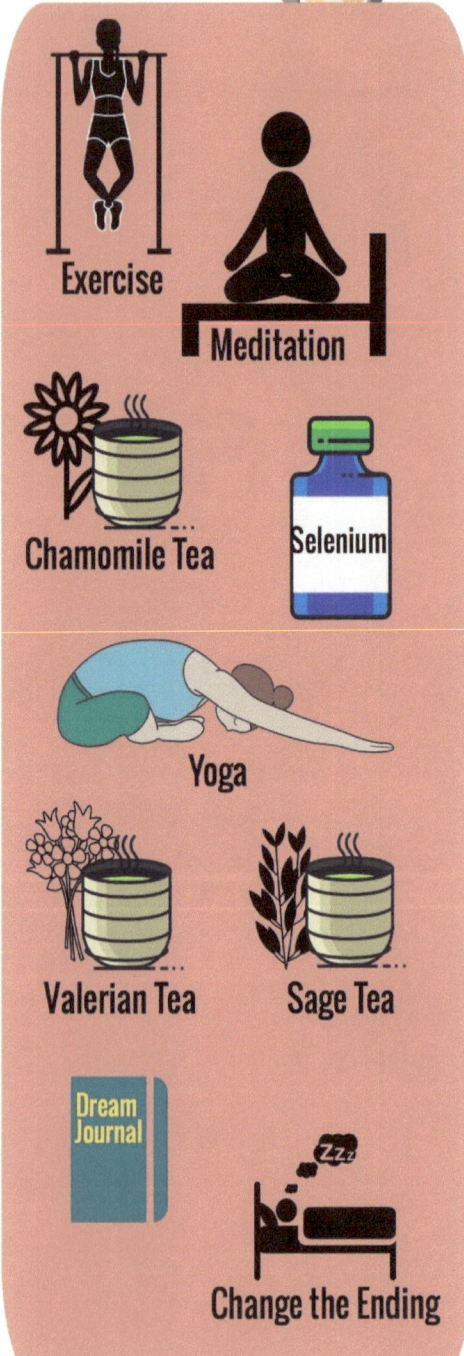

- NO Computer Before Bed
- Check Medication
- Cognitive Behavioral Therapy
- Relax
- Talk To Your Nightmare

- Exercise
- Meditation
- Chamomile Tea
- Selenium
- Yoga
- Valerian Tea
- Sage Tea
- Dream Journal
- Change the Ending

Oily Hair

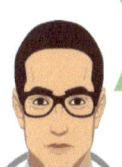
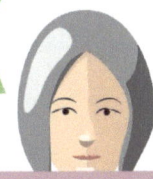
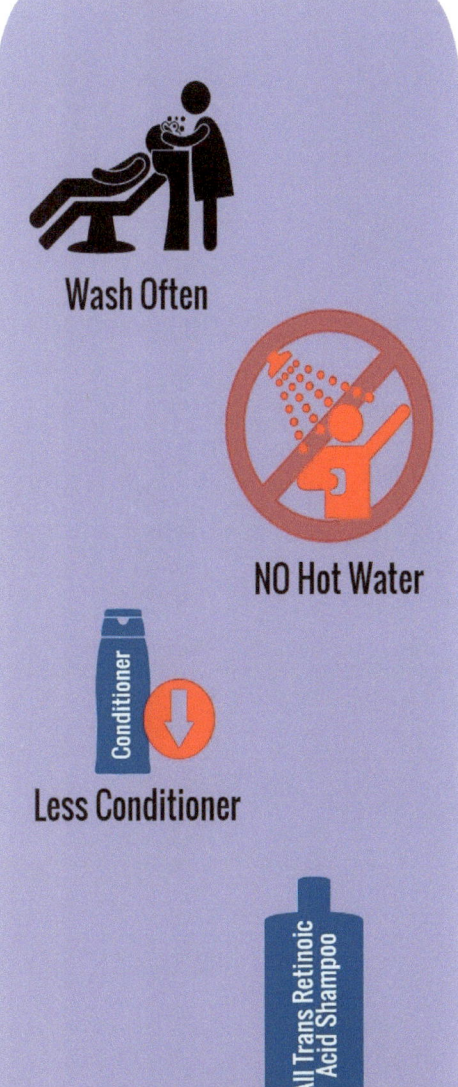
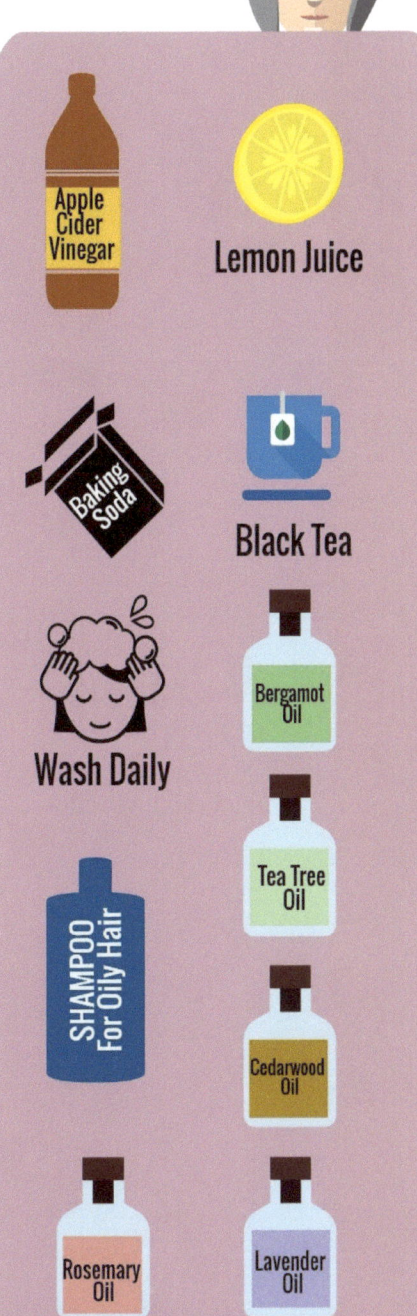

Oily Skin

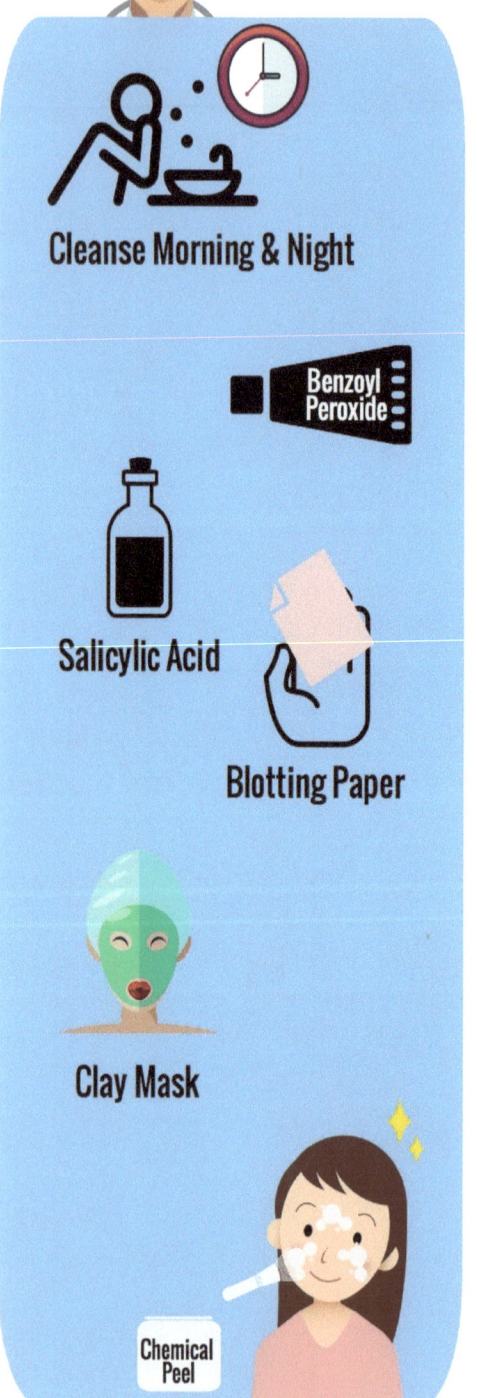
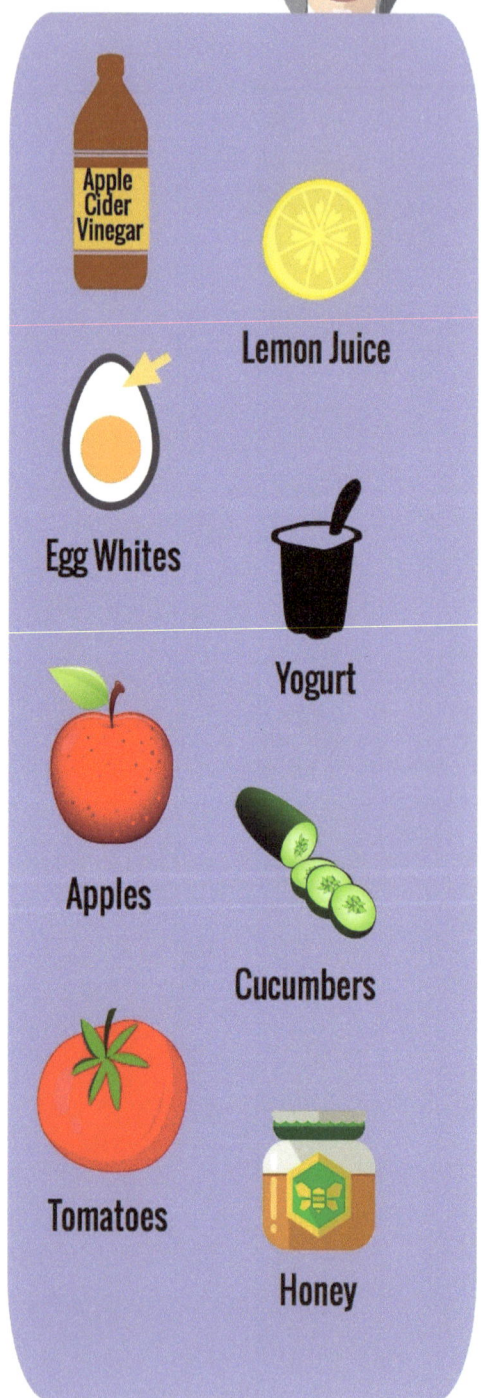

Osteoporosis

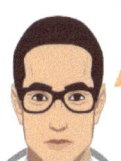
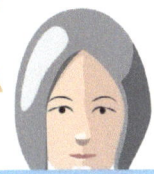
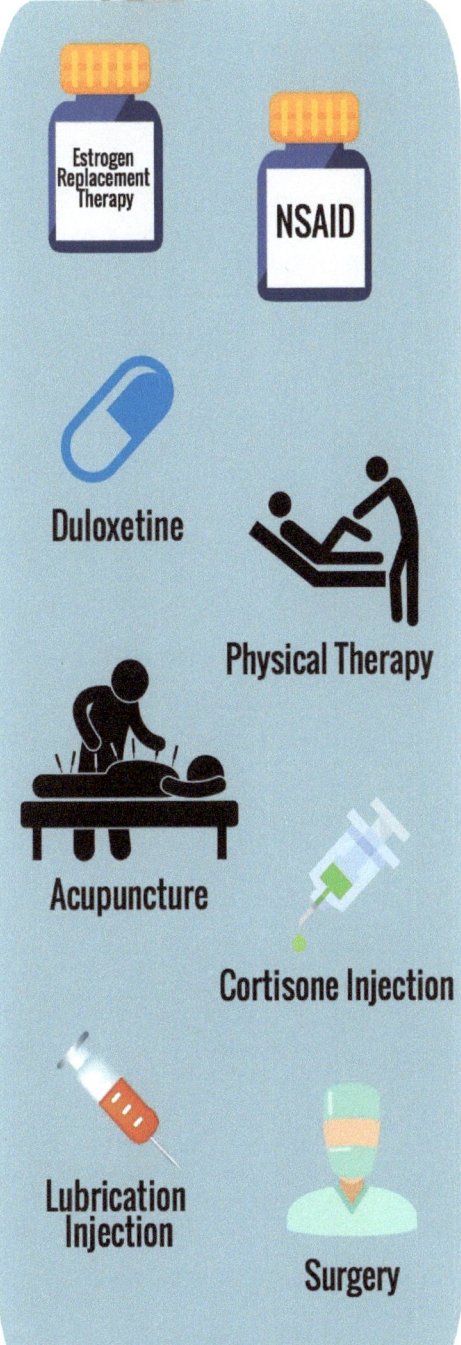
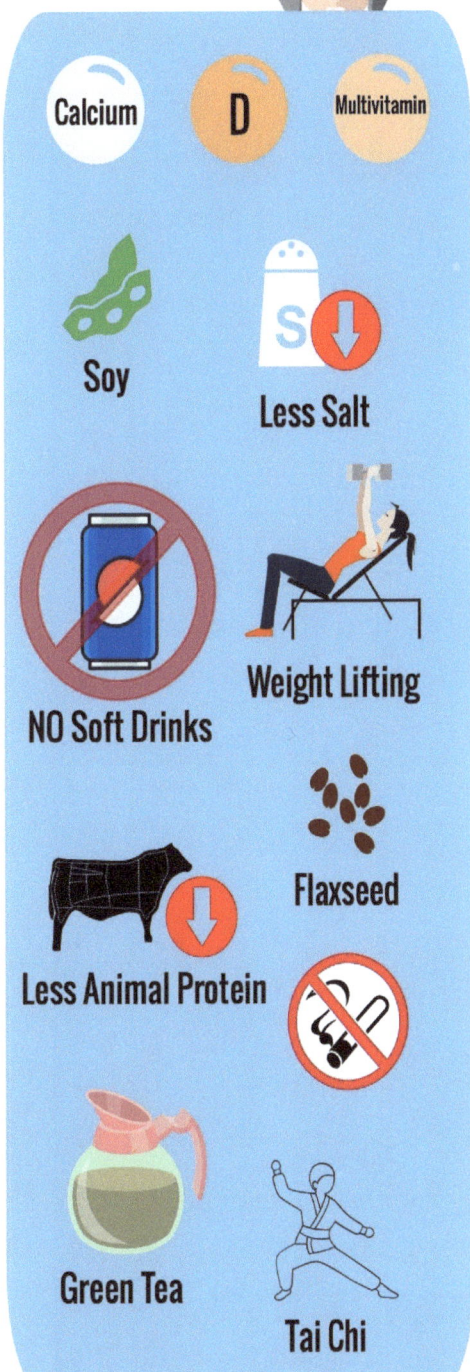

Obesity

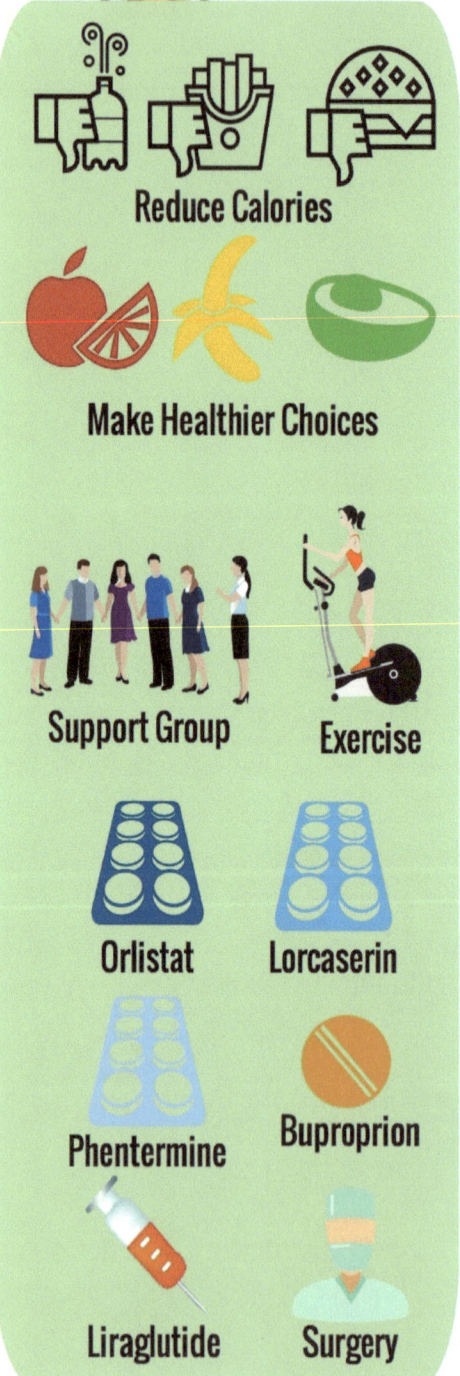
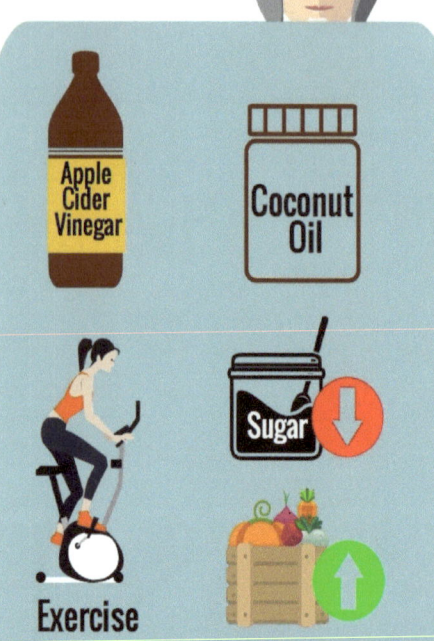
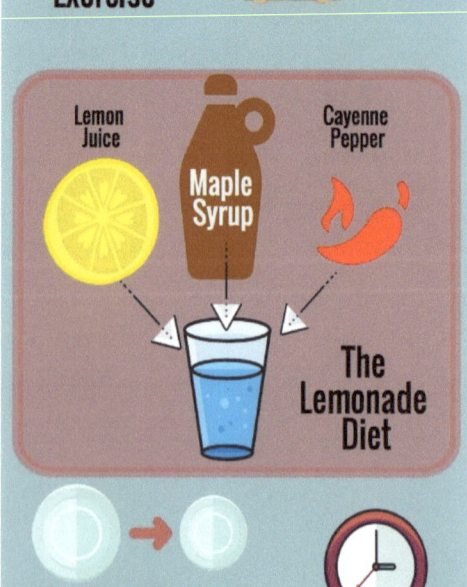

Panic Attacks

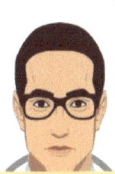 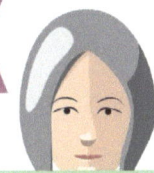

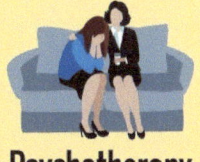
Psychotherapy

SSRI

SNRI

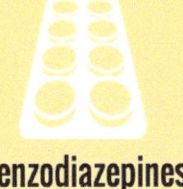
Benzodiazepines

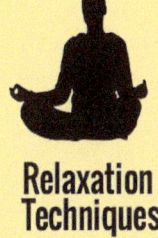
Relaxation Techniques

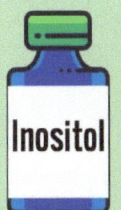
Inositol

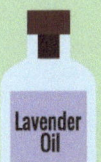
Lavender Oil

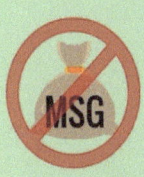
MSG

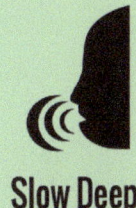
Slow Deep Breathing

Chat with Someone

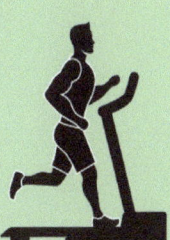

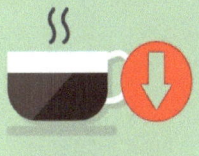

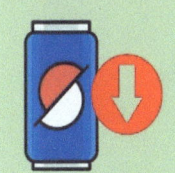

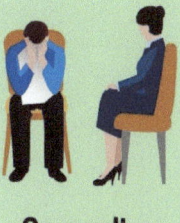
Counseling

Parkinson's Disease

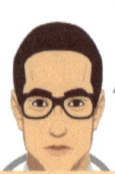
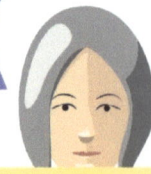

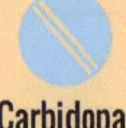
Carbidopa Levodopa

Dopamine Agonists

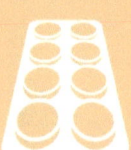
MAO Inhibitors

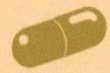
COMT Inhibitors

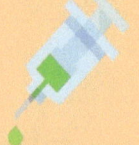
Anticholinergics

Amantadine

Exercise

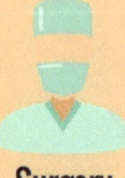
Surgery

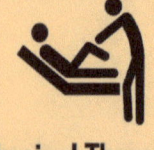
Physical Therapy

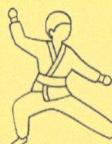
CoQ10

Tai Chi

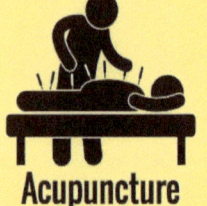
Acupuncture

Stretching

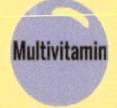
Multivitamin

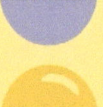
Fish Oil

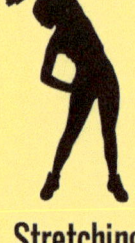
NO Processed Foods

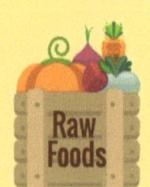
Raw Foods

NO Artificial Sweeteners

Pink Eye (Conjunctivitis)

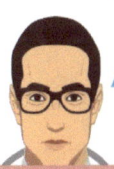
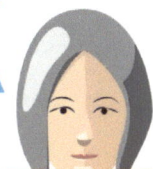

Medical Treatment

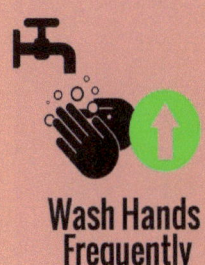
Wash Hands Frequently

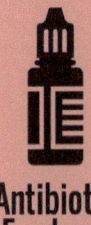
Antibiotic Eyedrops

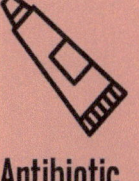
Antibiotic Ointment

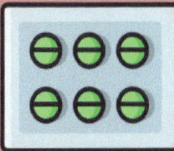
Antibiotics

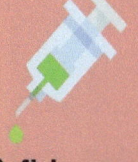
Ceftriaxone

Home Remedies

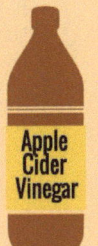
Apple Cider Vinegar

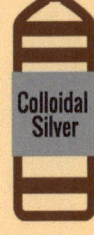
Colloidal Silver

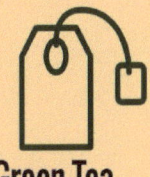
Green Tea Bag

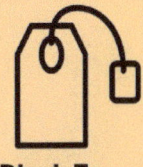
Black Tea Bag

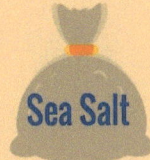
Sea Salt

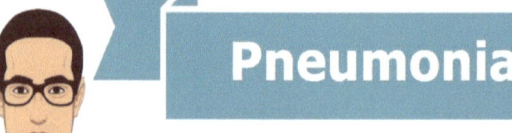

Pneumonia

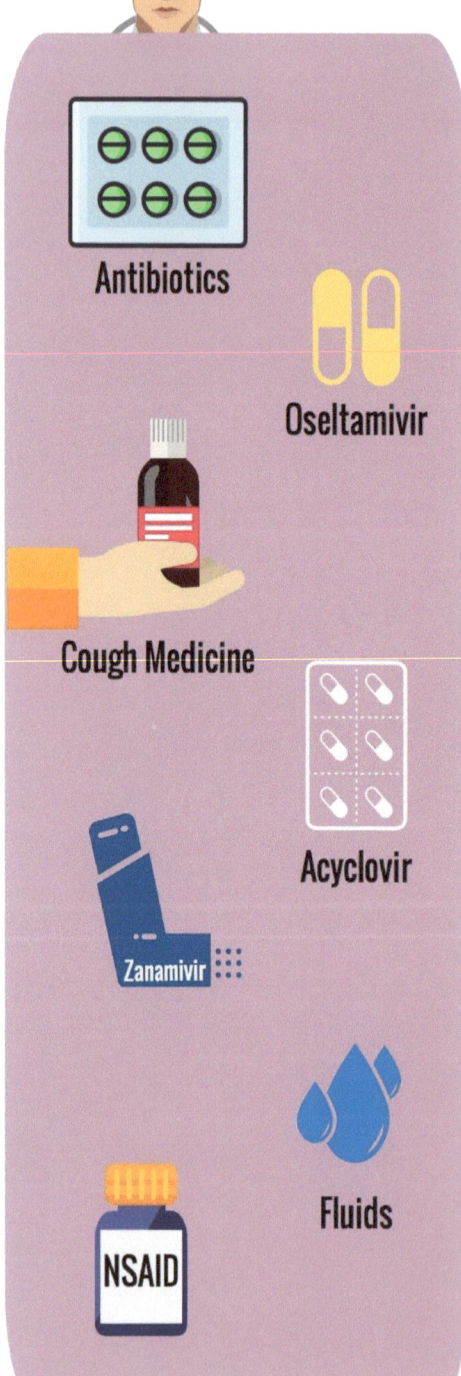
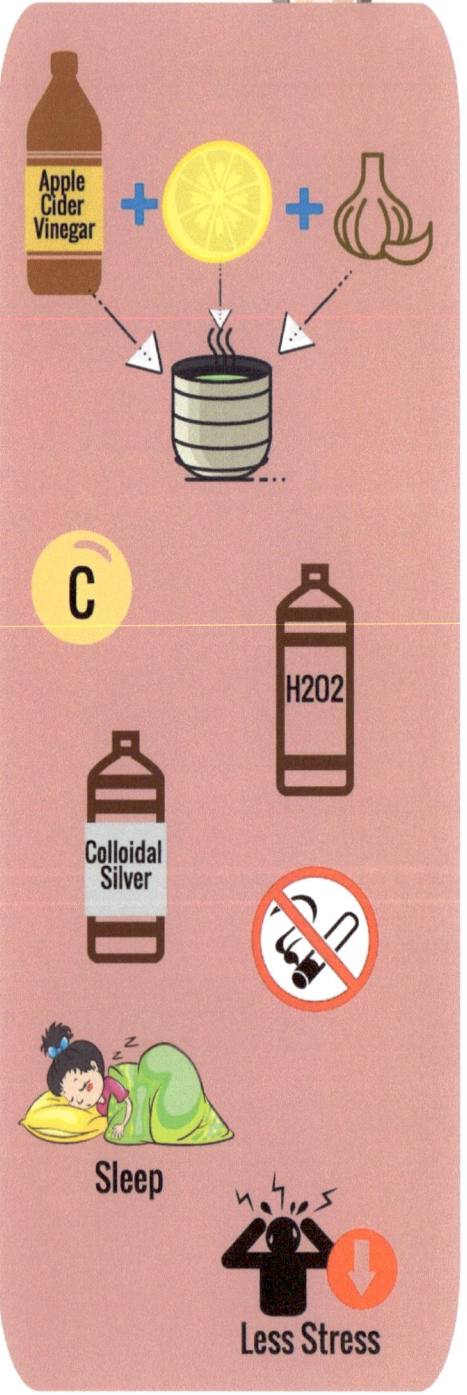

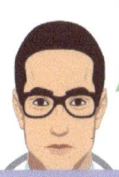 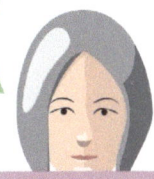

Premature Ejaculation

- The Kegel Exercise
- Climax Control Condom
- Anesthetic Cream
- SSRI
- PDE5 Inhibitor
- Counseling

- 5-HTP
- NO Porn
- Relaxation Techniques
- More Foreplay
- Fenugreek
- Ginkgo Biloba
- (reduce alcohol)
- (reduce smoking)

Premenstrual Syndrome

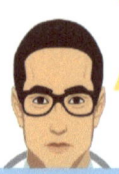
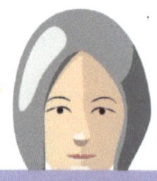
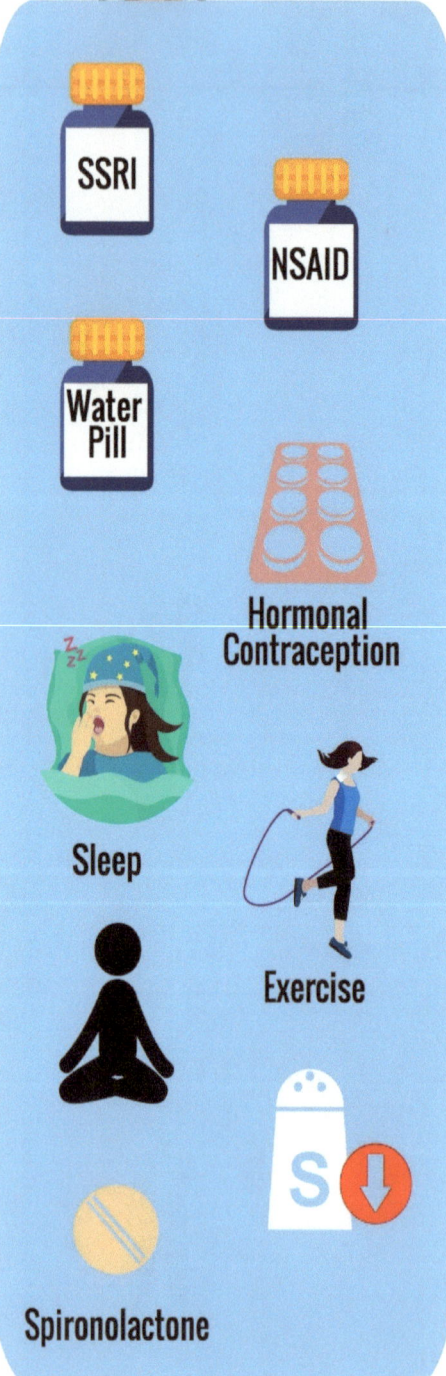
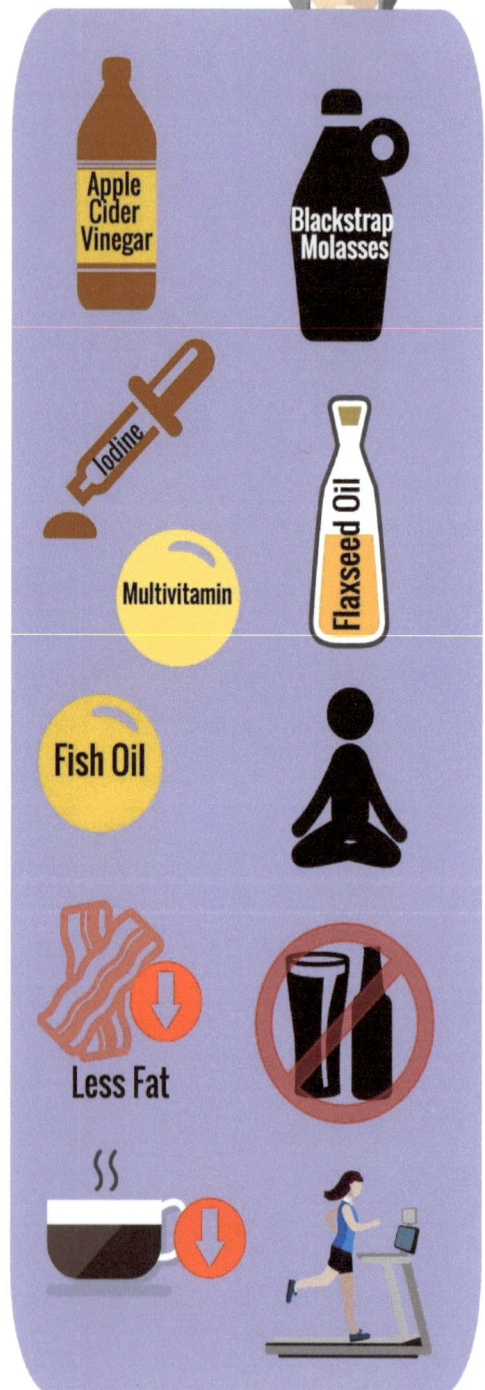

Prostate Problems

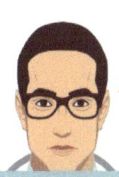
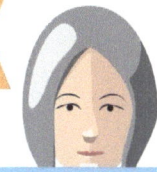

Medical Treatments

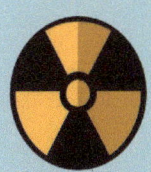
Radiation Therapy

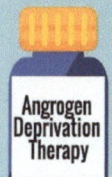
Androgen Deprivation Therapy

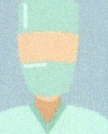
Surgery

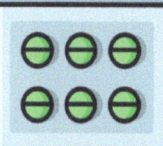
Antibiotics

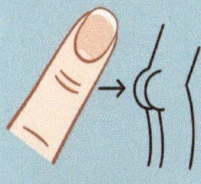
Drainage & Massage

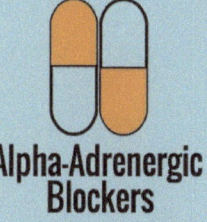
Alpha-Adrenergic Blockers

Natural Remedies

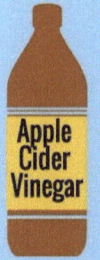
Apple Cider Vinegar

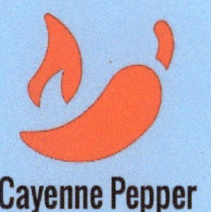
Cayenne Pepper

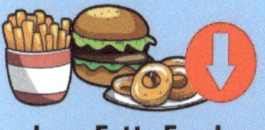
Less Fatty Foods

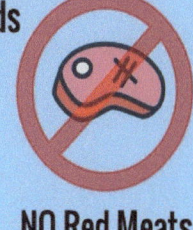
NO Red Meats

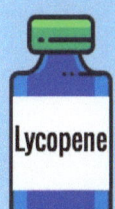
Lycopene

H2O2

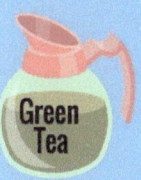
Green Tea

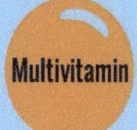
Multivitamin

Psoriasis

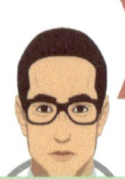
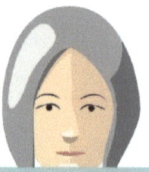
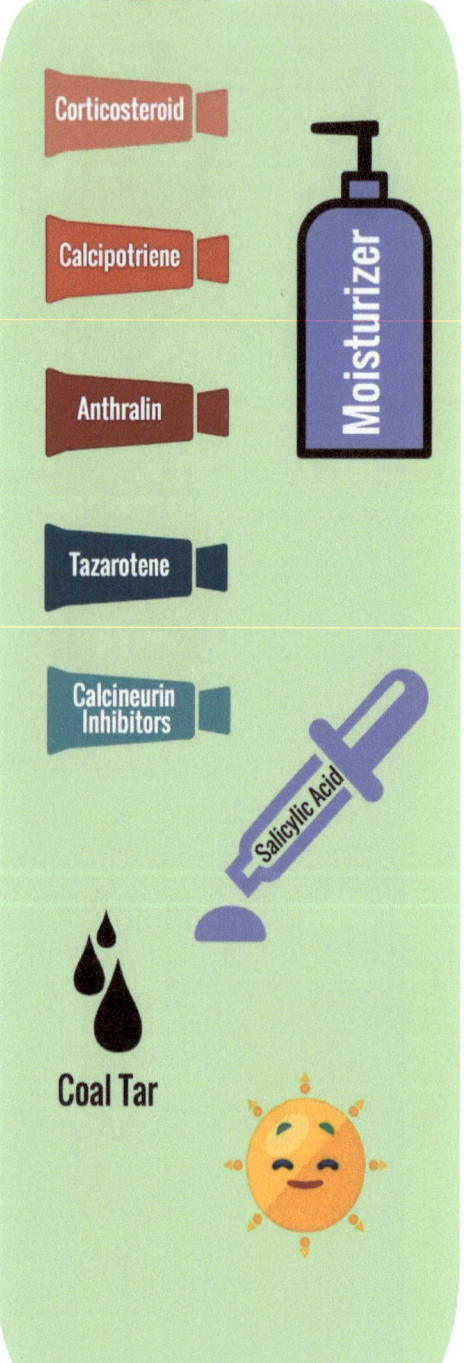
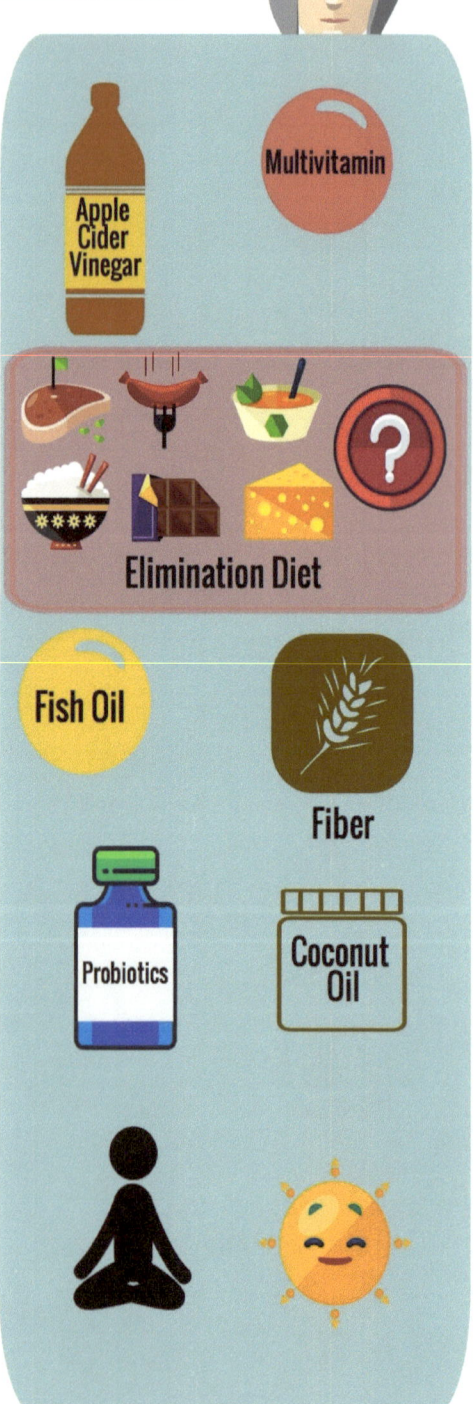

Rashes

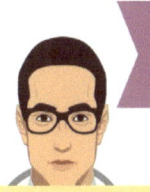
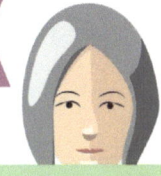

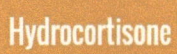
Hydrocortisone

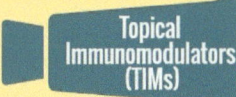
Topical Immunomodulators (TIMs)

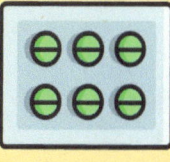
Antibiotics

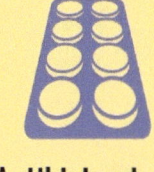
Antihistamines

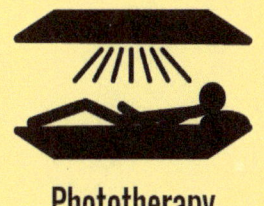
Phototherapy

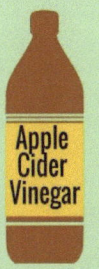
Apple Cider Vinegar

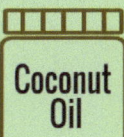
Coconut Oil

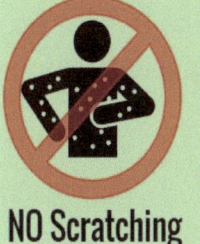
NO Scratching

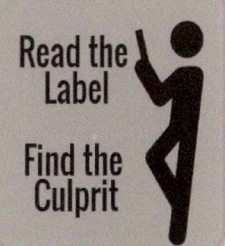
Read the Label
Find the Culprit

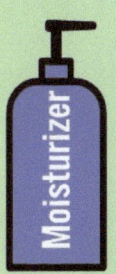
Moisturizer

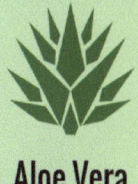
Aloe Vera

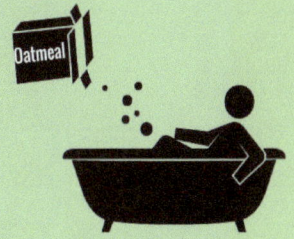
Oatmeal

Repetitive Strain Injury

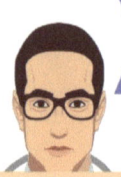
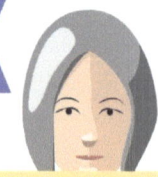

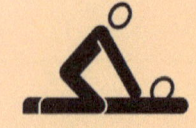
Physical Therapy

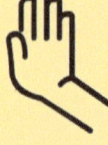
Stretch

NO Caffeine

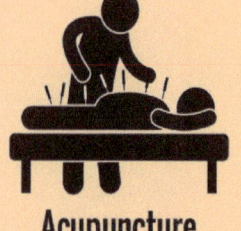
Acupuncture

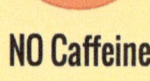 B

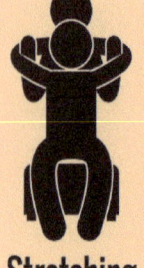
Stretching

Ice & Heat

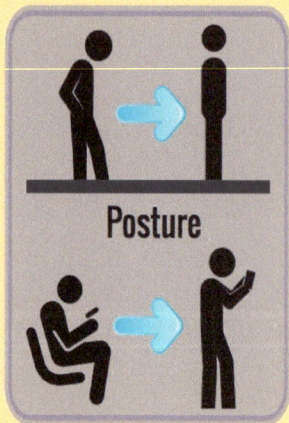
Posture

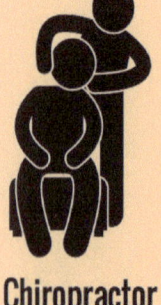
Chiropractor

NSAID

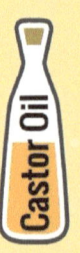
Castor Oil

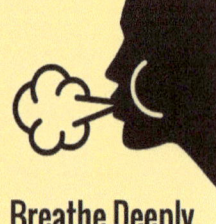
Breathe Deeply

Scars

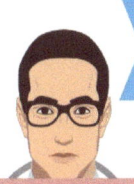 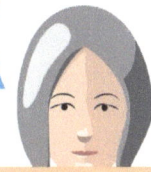

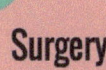
Surgery

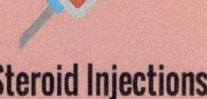
Steroid Injections

 E

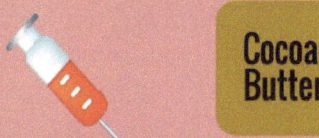
Filler Injections · Cocoa Butter

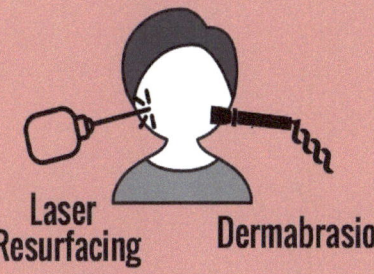
Laser Resurfacing · Dermabrasion

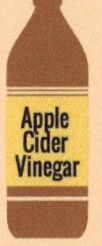
Apple Cider Vinegar

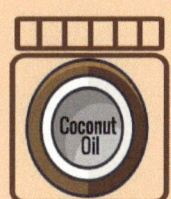
Coconut Oil

 E

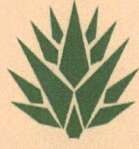
Aloe Vera

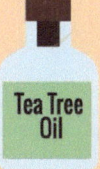
Tea Tree Oil

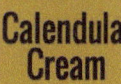
Calendula Cream

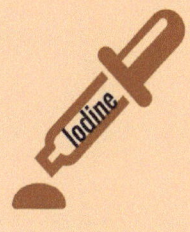
Iodine

Sciatica

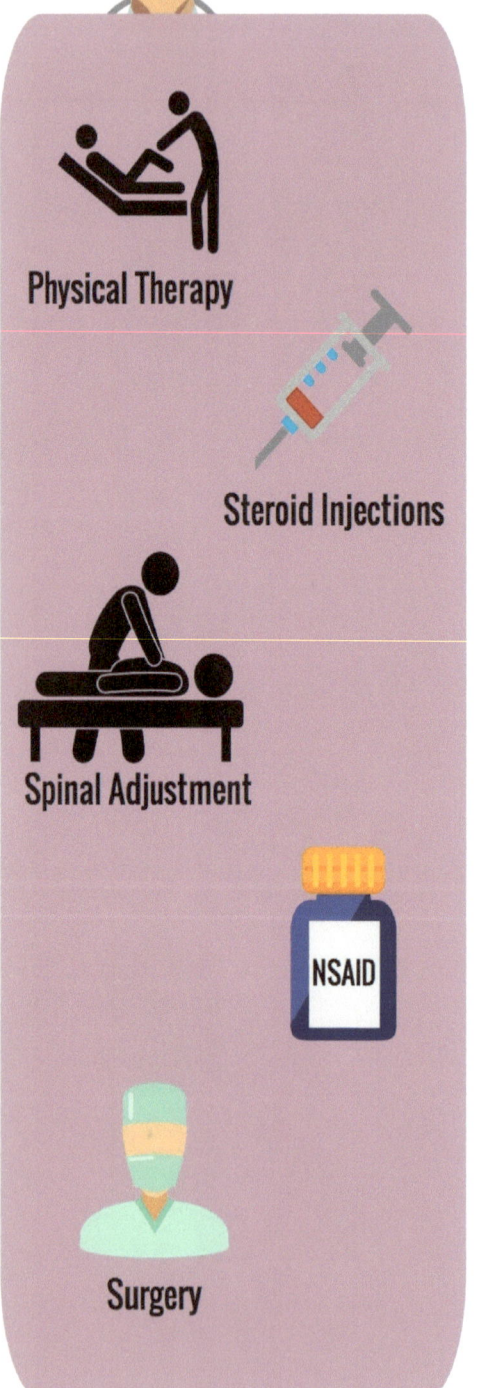
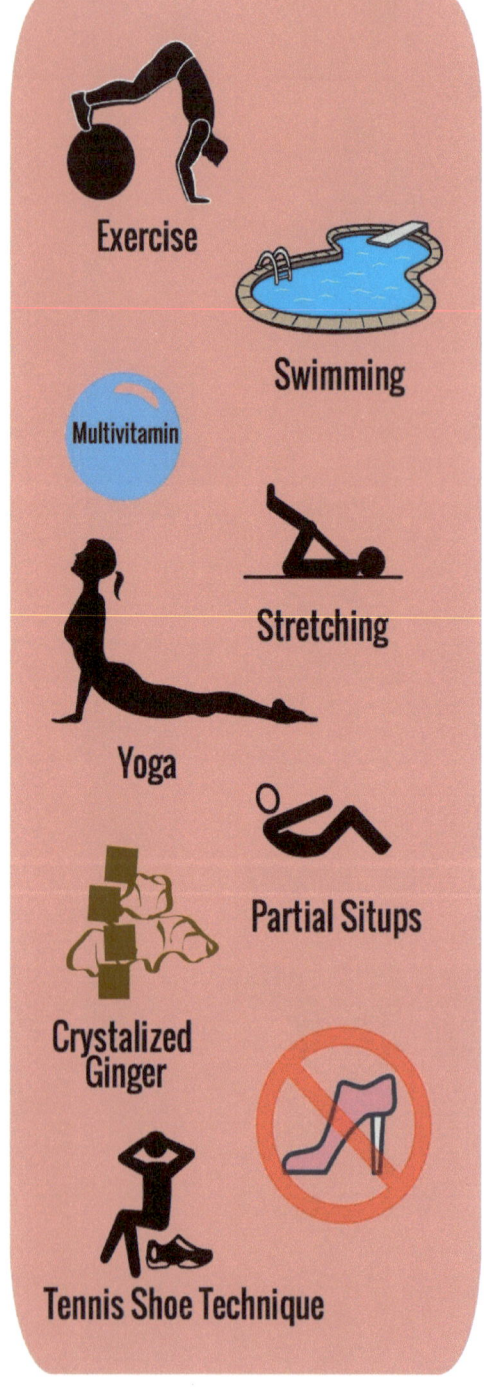

Sinusitis

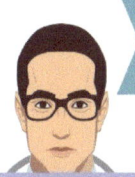
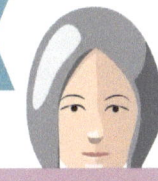

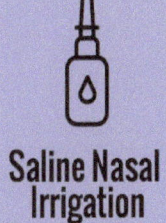
Saline Nasal Irrigation

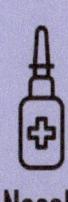
Nasal Corticosteroids

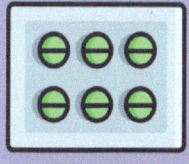
Antibiotics

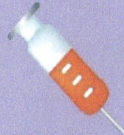
Allergy Shots

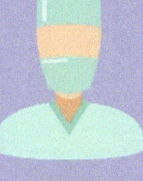
Surgery

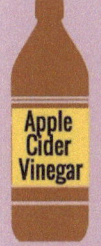
Apple Cider Vinegar

Cayenne Pepper

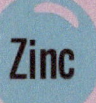
Zinc

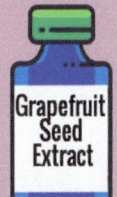
Grapefruit Seed Extract

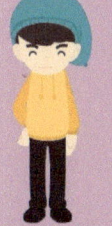
Keep Head Warm

Fluids

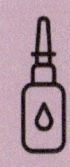
Saline Nasal Spray

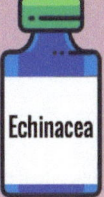
Echinacea

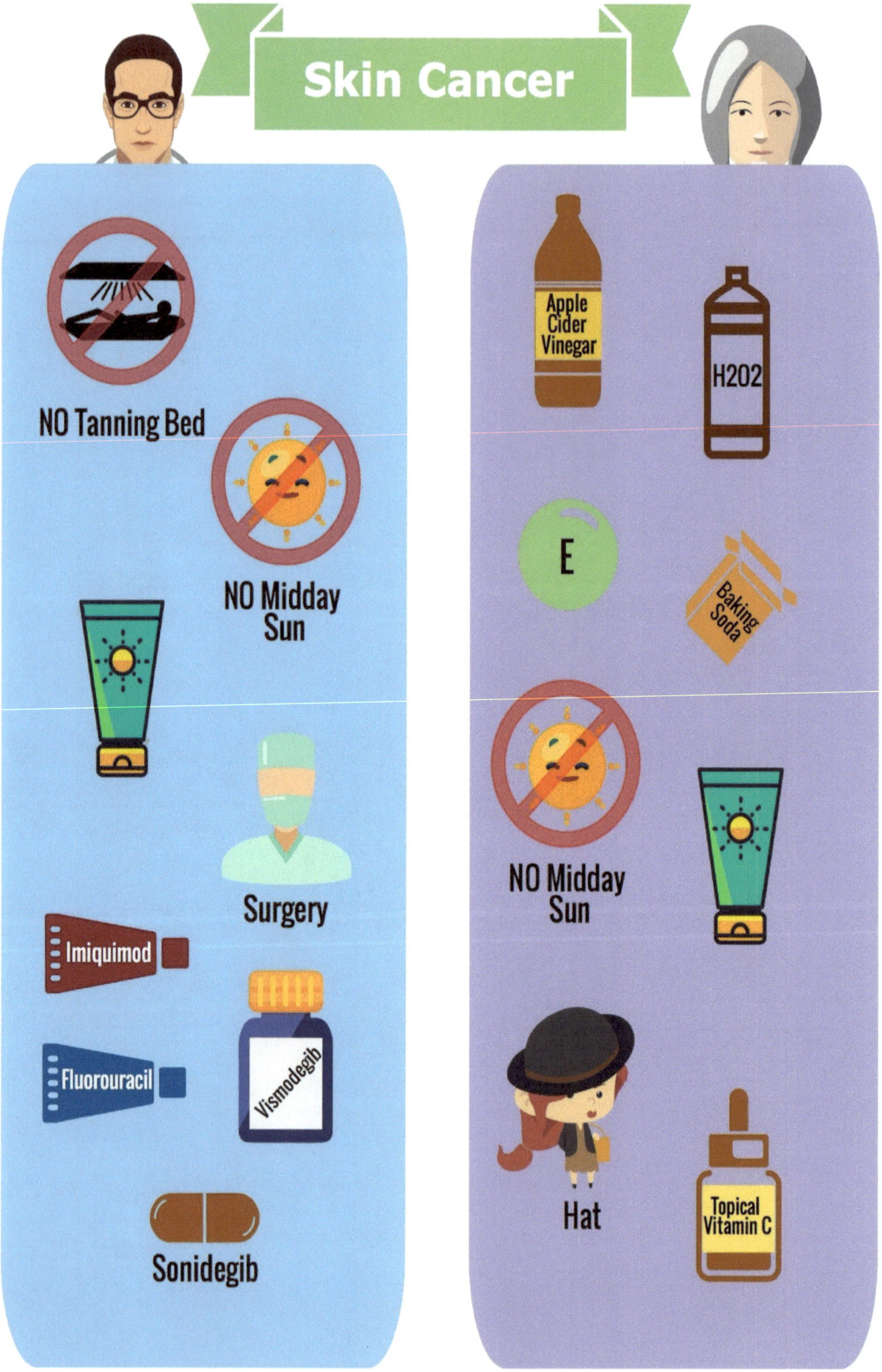

Skin Cancer

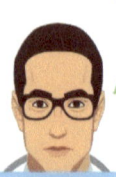
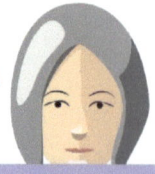
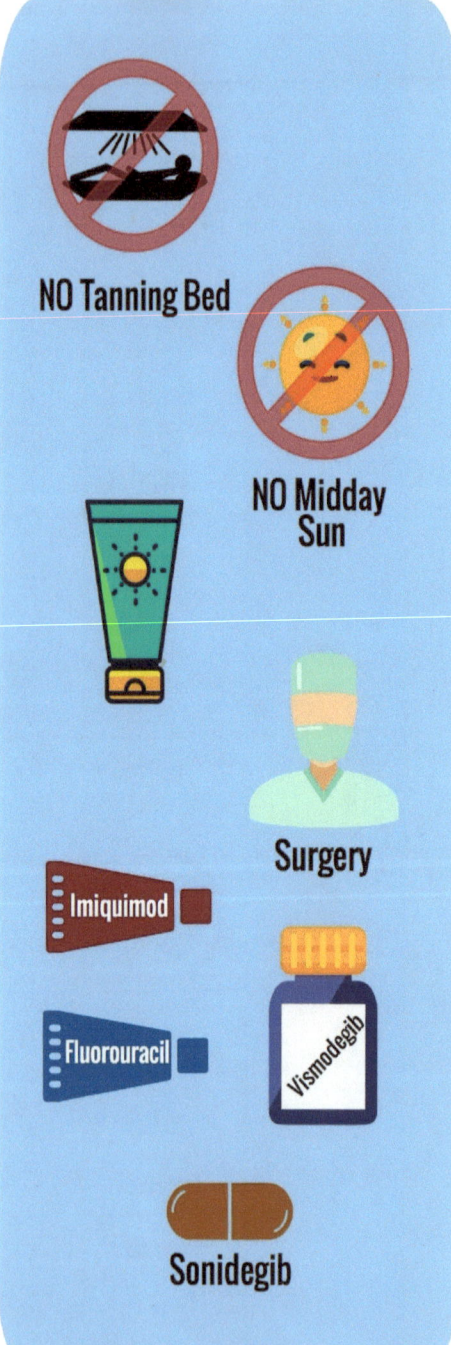

- NO Tanning Bed
- NO Midday Sun
- Surgery
- Imiquimod
- Fluorouracil
- Vismodegib
- Sonidegib

- Apple Cider Vinegar
- H2O2
- E
- Baking Soda
- NO Midday Sun
- Hat
- Topical Vitamin C

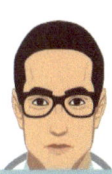 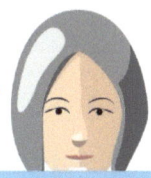

Sleep Apnea

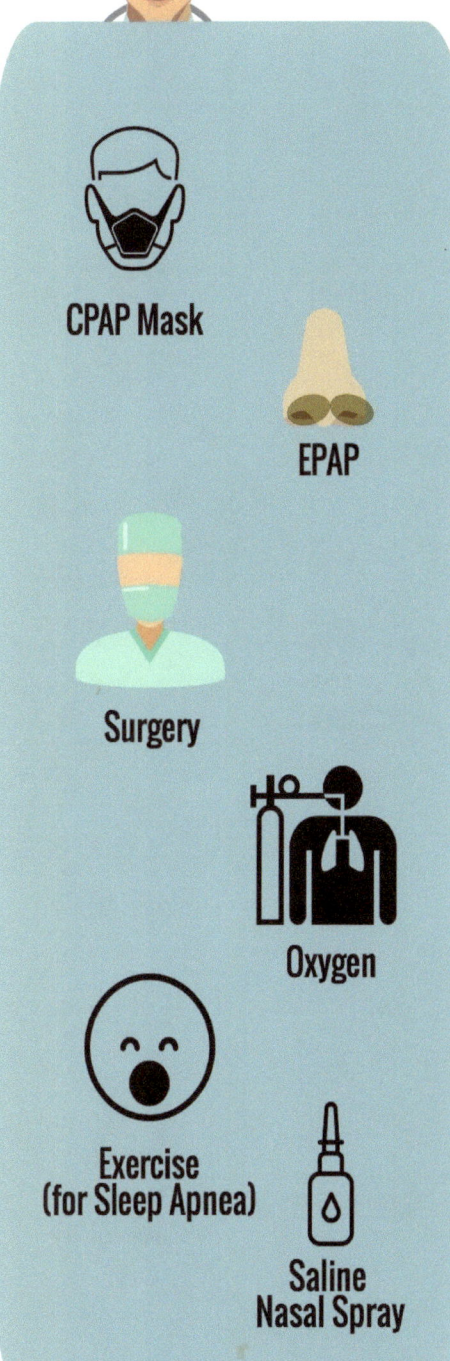
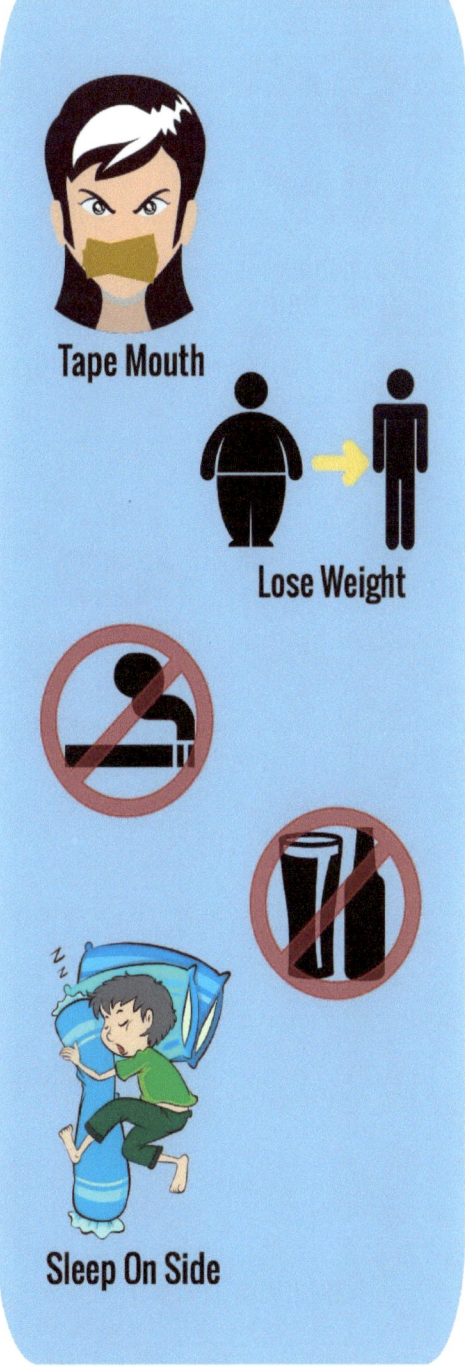

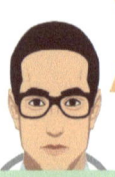 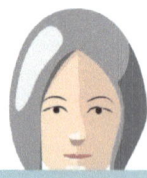

Snoring

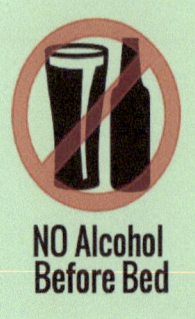
NO Alcohol Before Bed

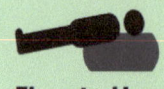
Elevate Head

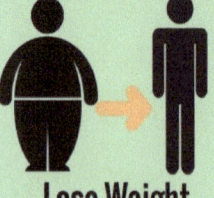
Lose Weight

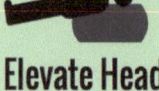
Mandibular Advancement Splints

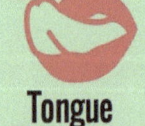
Tongue Retaining Device

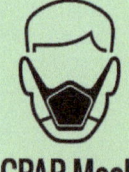
CPAP Mask

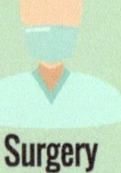
Surgery

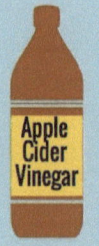 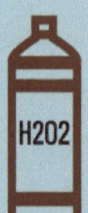

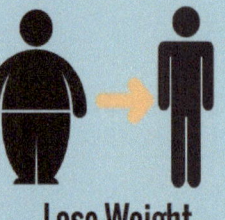
Lose Weight

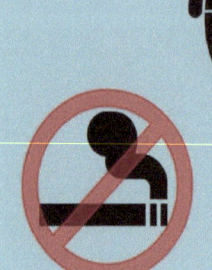

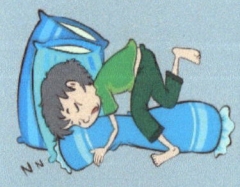
Elevated Bed

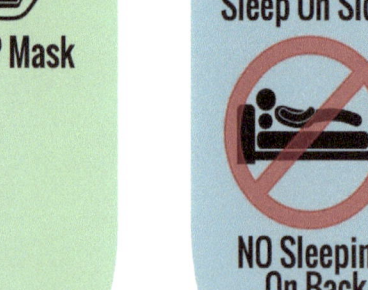
Sleep On Side

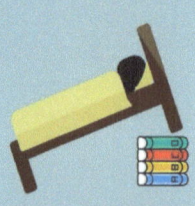
Essential Oil Throat Spray

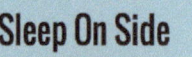

NO Sleeping On Back

Sore Throat

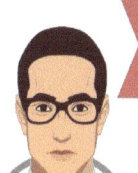
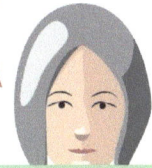

Conventional

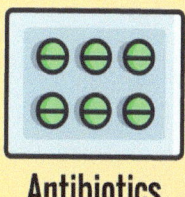
Antibiotics

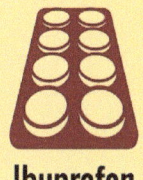
Ibuprofen

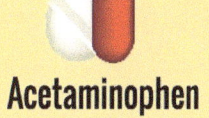
Acetaminophen

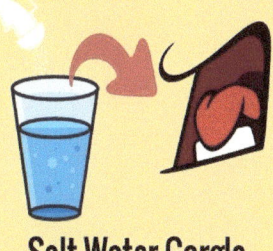
Salt Water Gargle

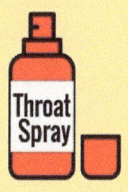
Throat Spray

Natural

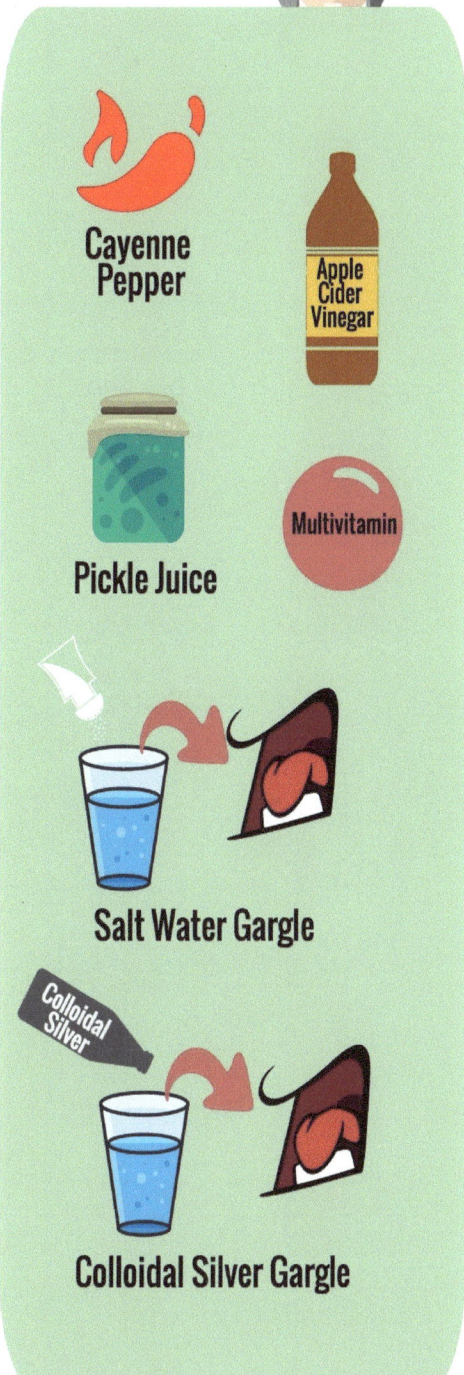

- Cayenne Pepper
- Apple Cider Vinegar
- Pickle Juice
- Multivitamin
- Salt Water Gargle
- Colloidal Silver Gargle

Stomach Pain

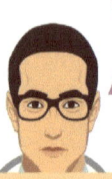
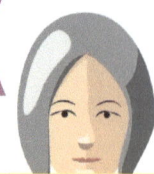

Simethicone

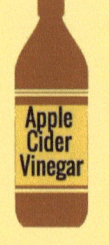
H-2 Receptor Blockers

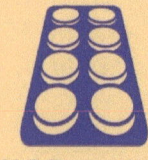
Apple Cider Vinegar

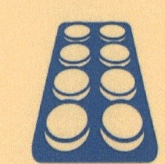
Proton Pump Inhibitors

Turmeric

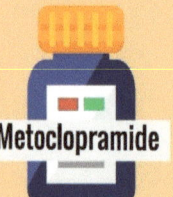
Metoclopramide

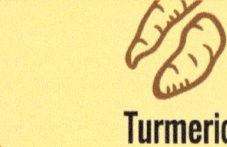
Baking Soda

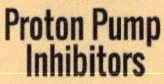
SSRI

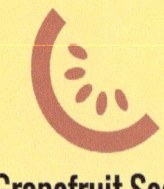
Grapefruit Seed Extract

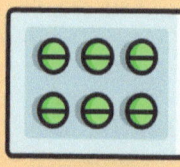
Antibiotics

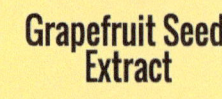
Garlic

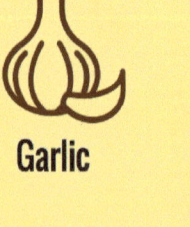
NSAID

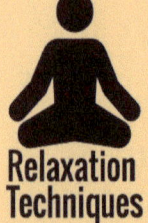
Relaxation Techniques

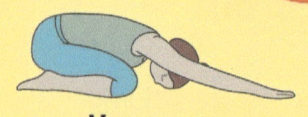
Yoga

Stomach Cancer

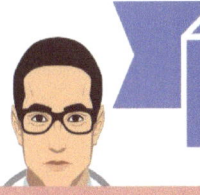
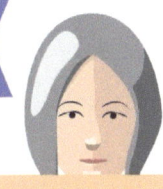

Medical Treatments

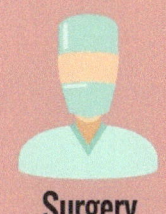
Surgery

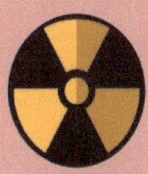
Radiation Therapy

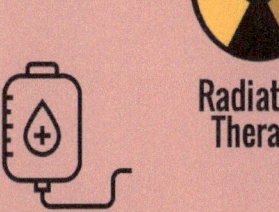
Chemotherapy

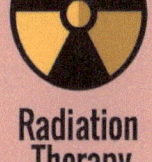
Trastuzumab

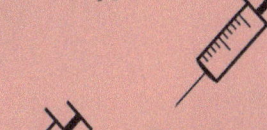
Ramucirumab

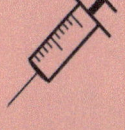
Imatinib

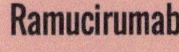
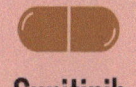
Sunitinib

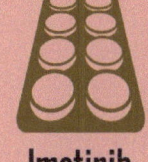
Regorafenib

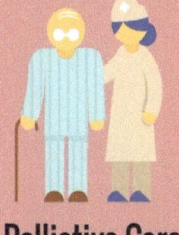
Palliative Care

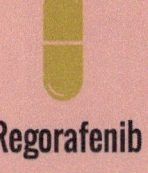

Diet & Lifestyle

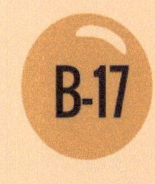
B-17

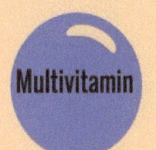
Multivitamin

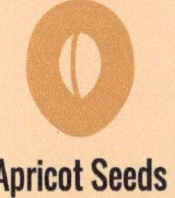
Apricot Seeds

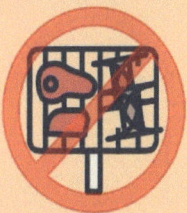
NO Overcooked Meats

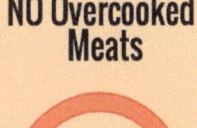
Fruits & Vegetables

NO Salt

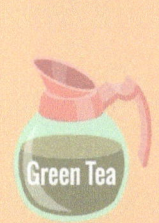
Green Tea

NO Smoking

NO Preserved Foods

NO Alcohol

Stress
Exercise
Meditation
Sense Of Humor
Socialize
Hobbies
Sleep
5-HTP
Rhodiola
B Complex
Exercise
Ginseng
Nature
Lavender Oil
NO Multitasking

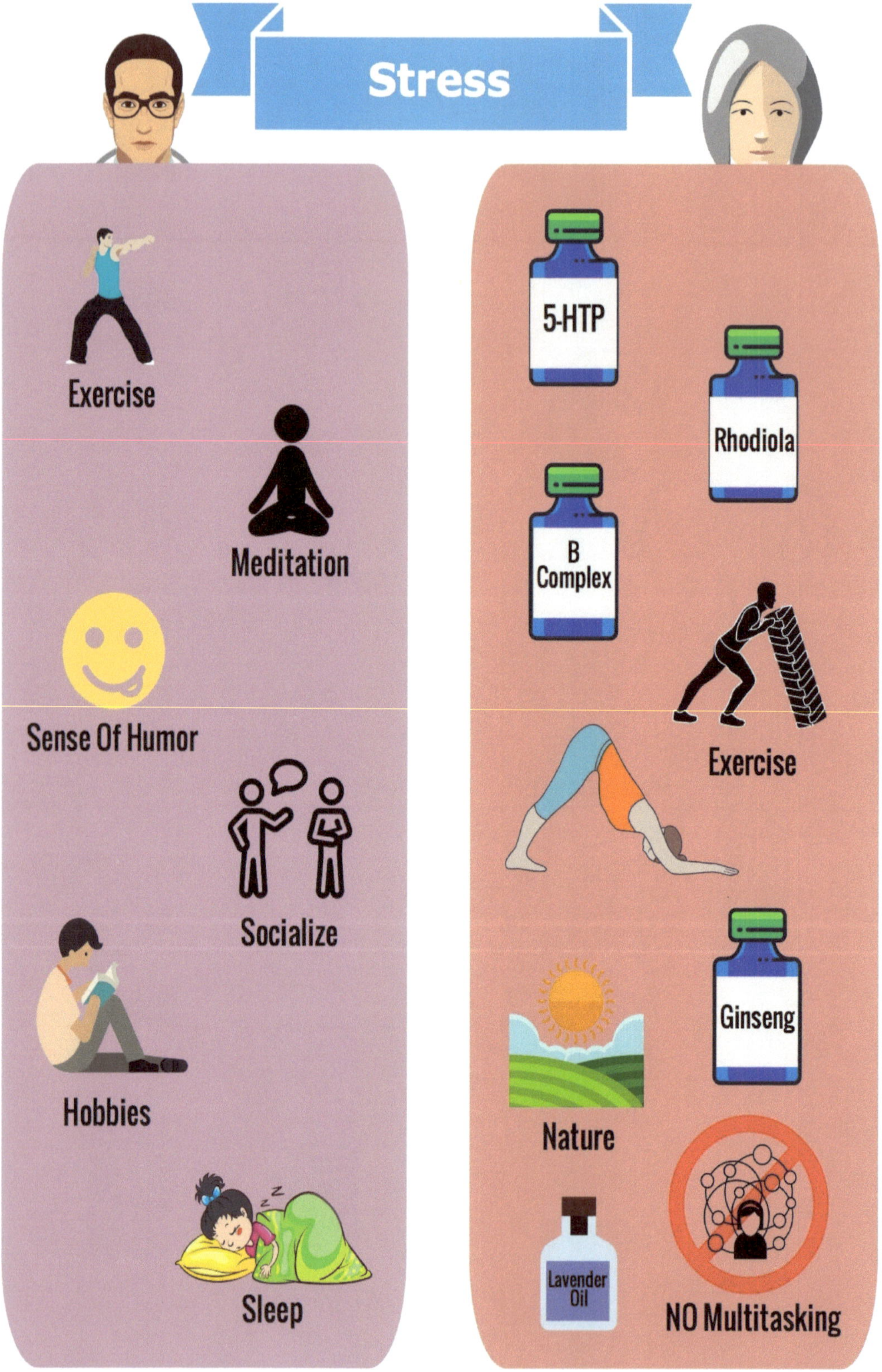

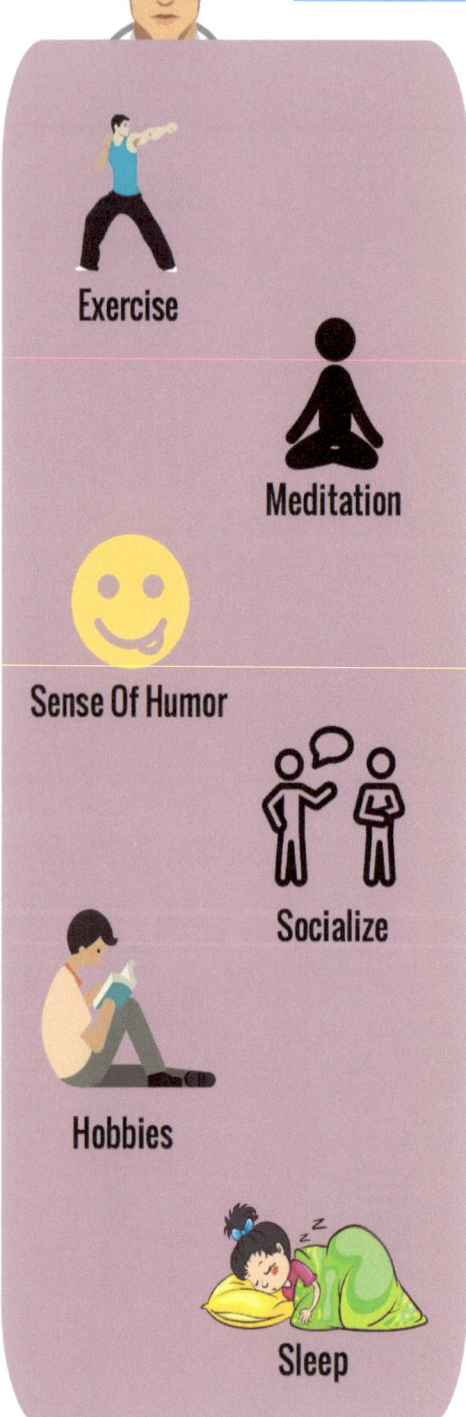

Stroke

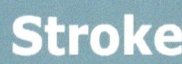
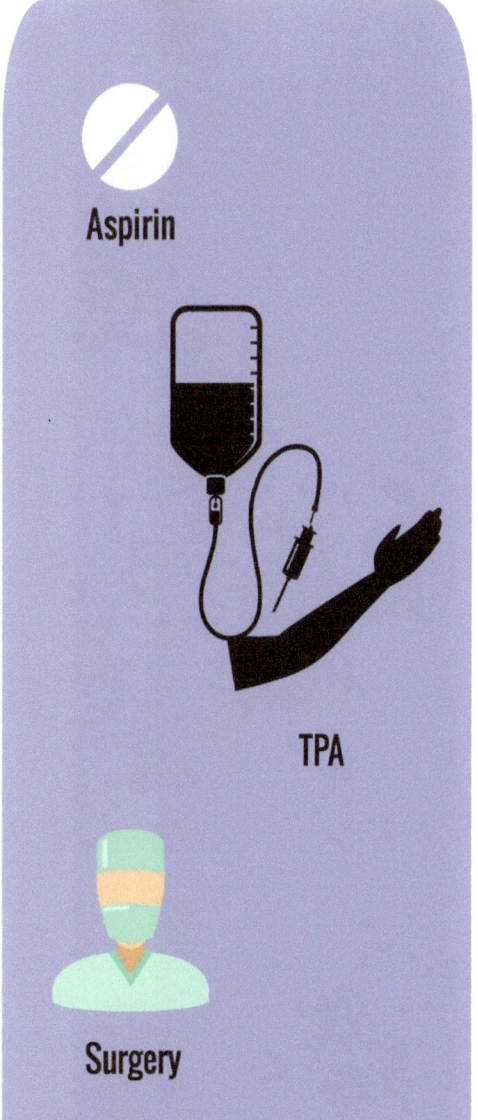
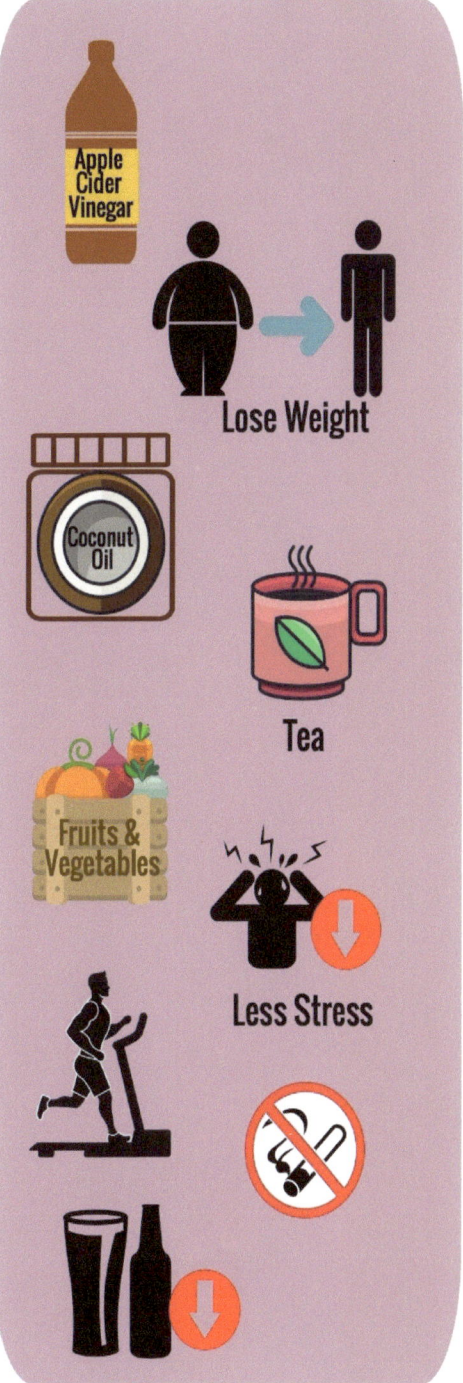

Tooth Sensitivity

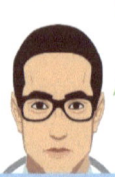
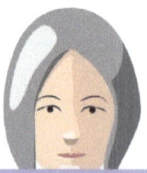

- Desensitizing Toothpaste
- Fluoride
- Gum Graft / Root Canal
- (No soda)

- Soft Bristles
- Baking Soda
- Oil Pulling (Coconut Oil)
- H2O2
- Magnesium
- Black Walnut
- Apple
- Floss

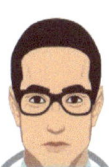 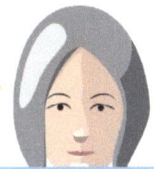

Tooth Stains

- Whitening Toothpaste
- Whitening Strips
- Carbamide Peroxide
- H2O2

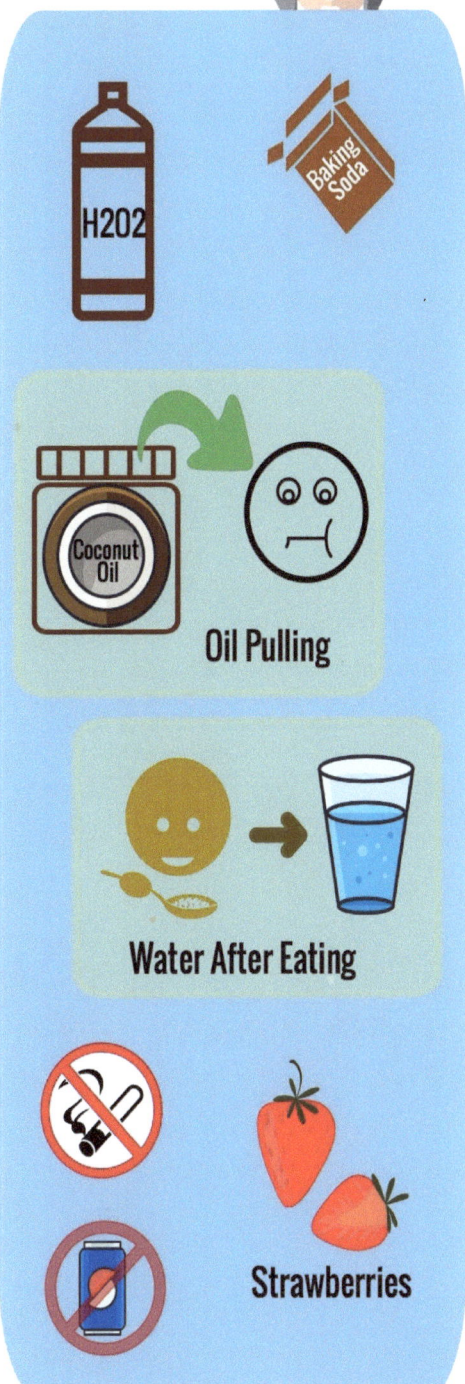

- H2O2
- Baking Soda
- Oil Pulling
- Water After Eating
- (No smoking)
- (No soda)
- Strawberries

Tumors

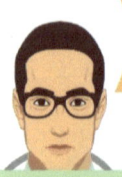 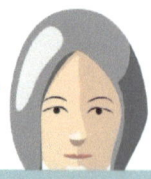

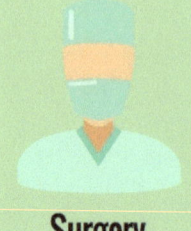
Surgery

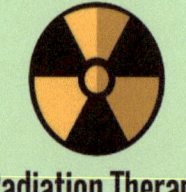
Radiation Therapy

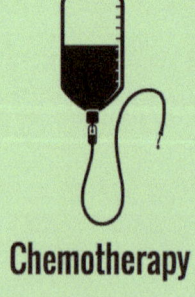
Chemotherapy

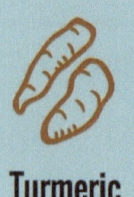 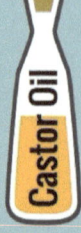
Turmeric   **Castor Oil**

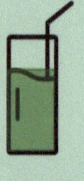 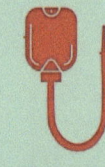
The Gerson Therapy

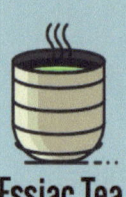 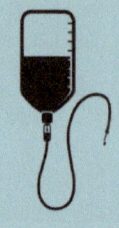
Essiac Tea   **Chelation Therapy**

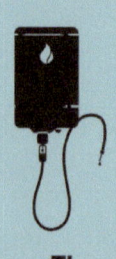 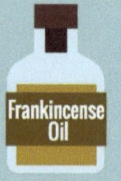
Ozone Therapy   **Frankincense Oil**

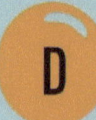

Ulcer

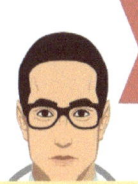
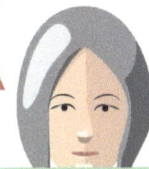

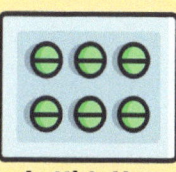
Antibiotics

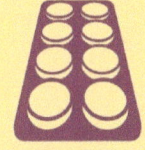
Proton Pump Inhibitors

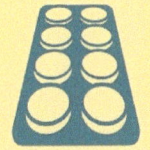
H-2 Blockers

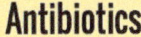
Antacid

Sucralfate

Isoprostol

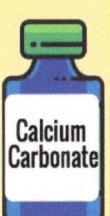
Calcium Carbonate

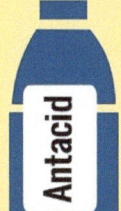

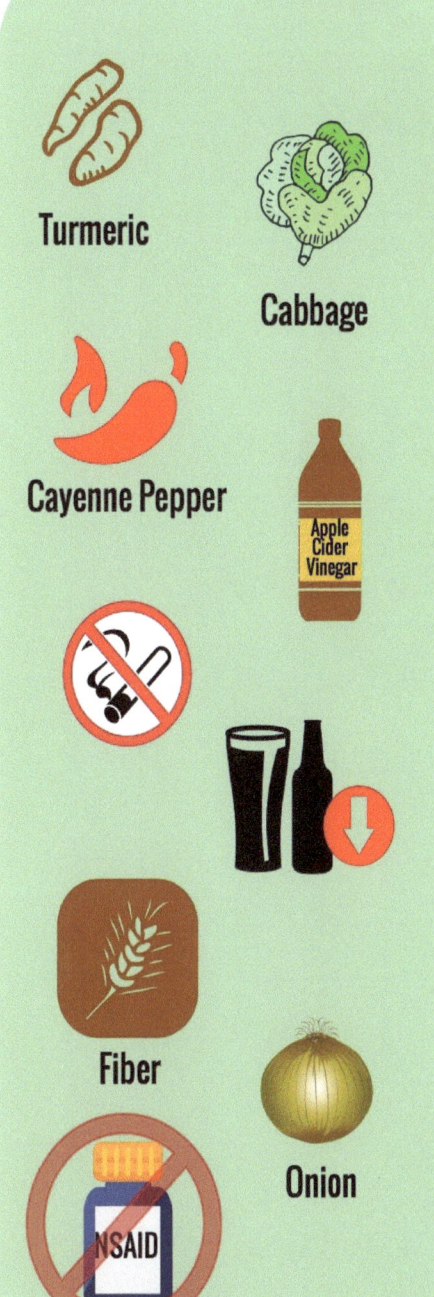

Turmeric

Cabbage

Cayenne Pepper

Apple Cider Vinegar

Fiber

Onion

NSAID

Urinary Tract Infection

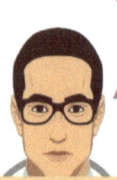
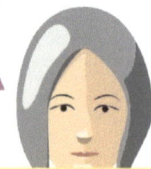

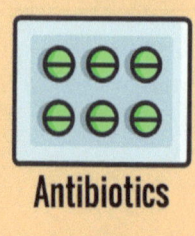
Antibiotics

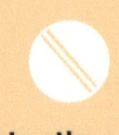
Trimethoprim

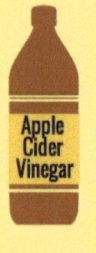
Apple Cider Vinegar

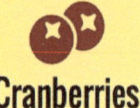
Cranberries

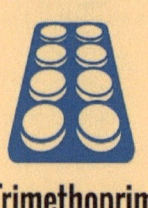
Trimethoprim

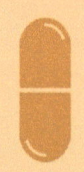
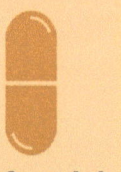
Nitrofurantoin

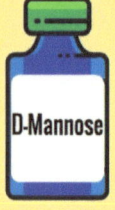
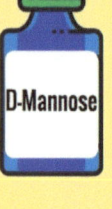
D-Mannose

Baking Soda

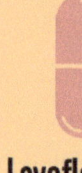
Ciprofloxacin

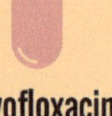
Levofloxacin

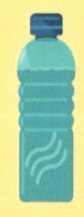

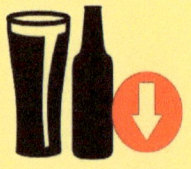

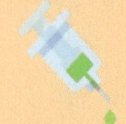
Cephalexin

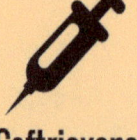
Ceftriaxone

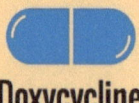

Azithromycin **Doxycycline**

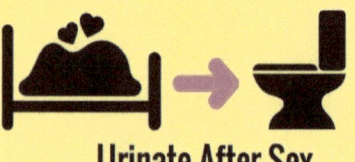
Urinate After Sex

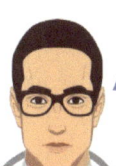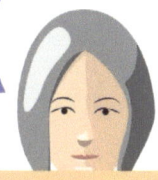

Varicose Veins

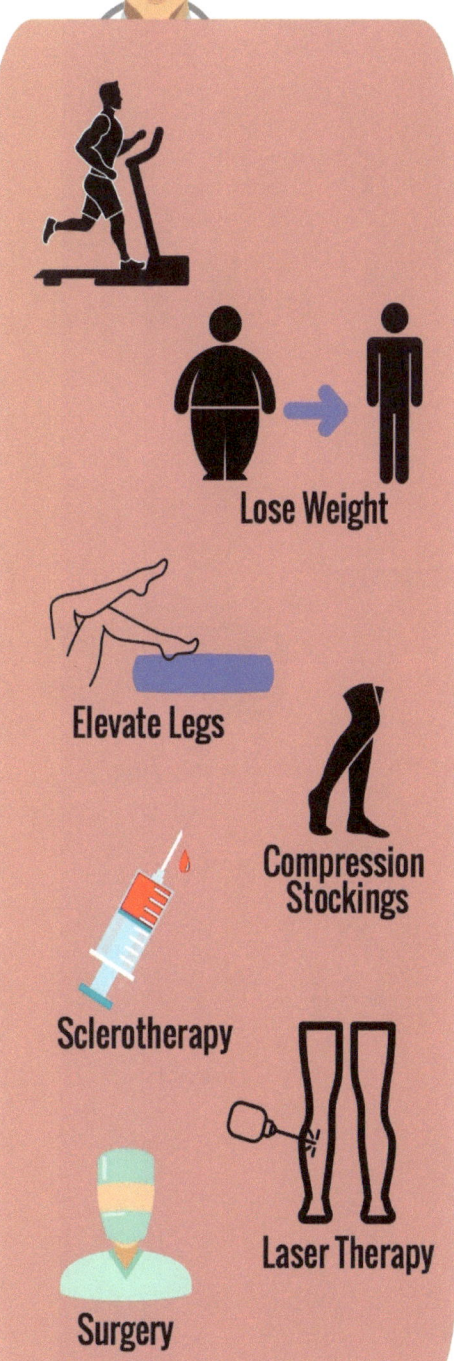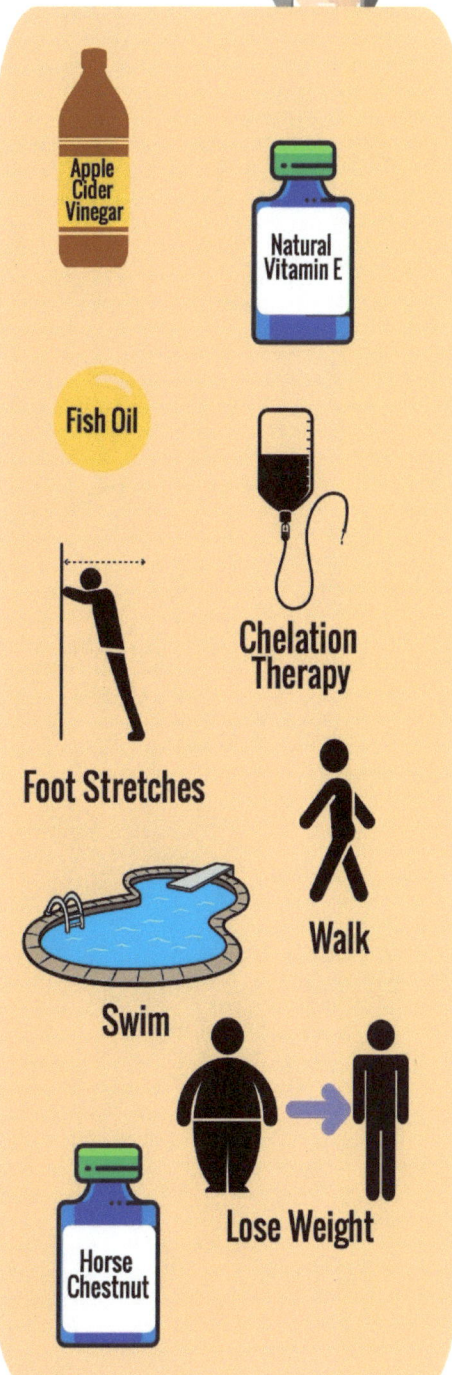

Vision Problems

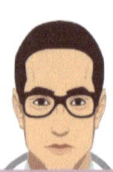
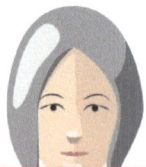

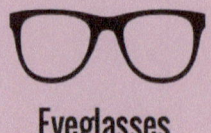
Eyeglasses

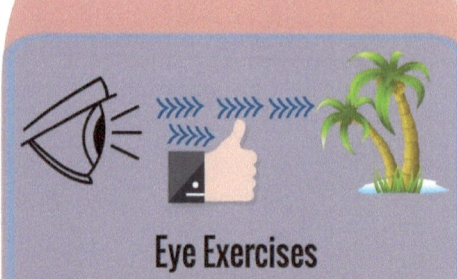
Eye Exercises

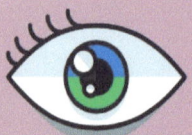
Contact Lenses

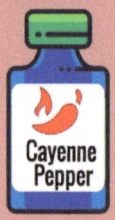
Cayenne Pepper

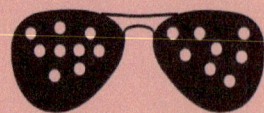
Pinhole Glasses

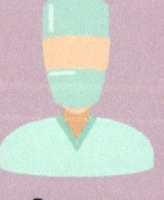
Surgery

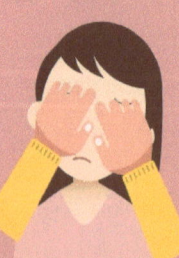
Palming

Wart

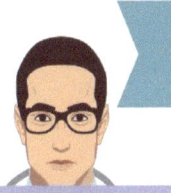
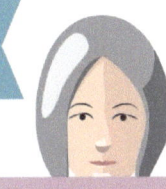

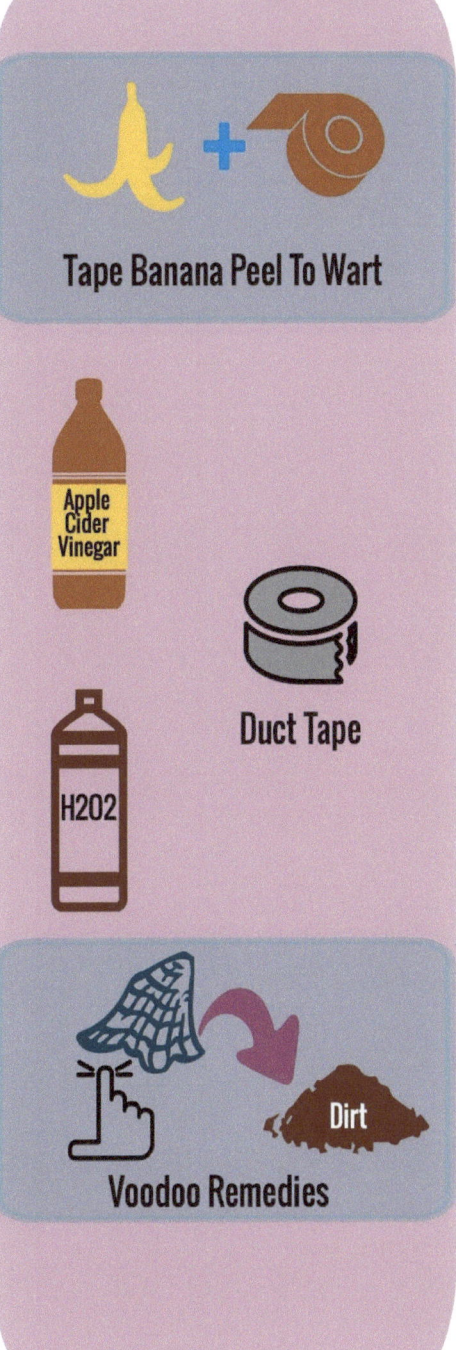

Water Retention

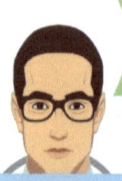
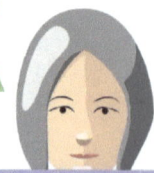

- Less Salt
- Healthy Diet
- Check Medication

- Apple Cider Vinegar
- Garlic
- NO "Added Salt" Foods
- B6
- Elevate Feet
- Support Hose

Wrinkles

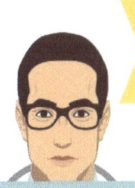
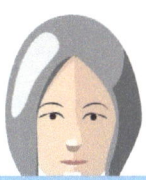
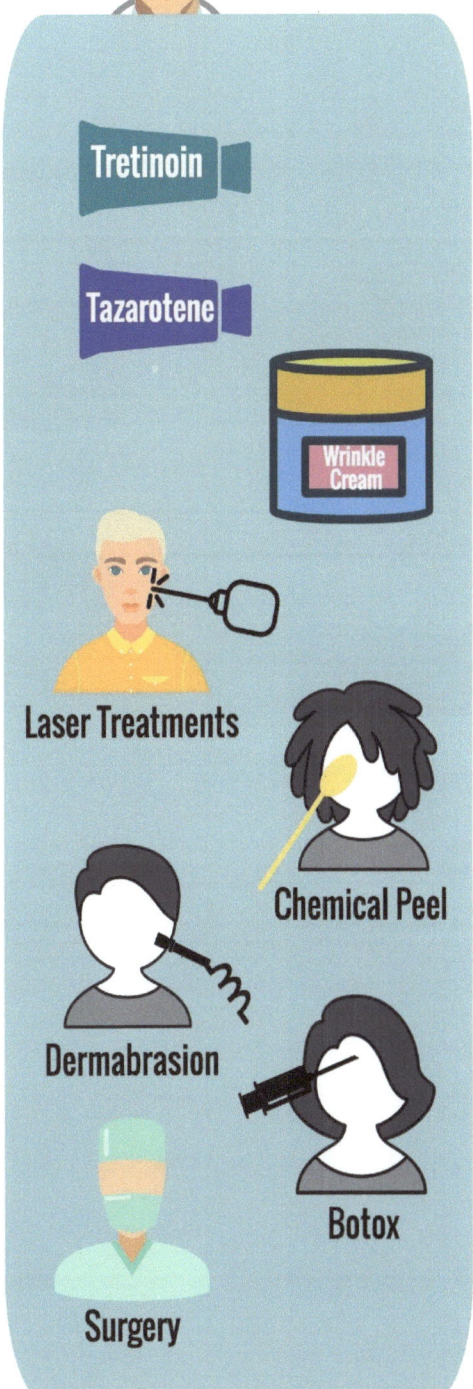
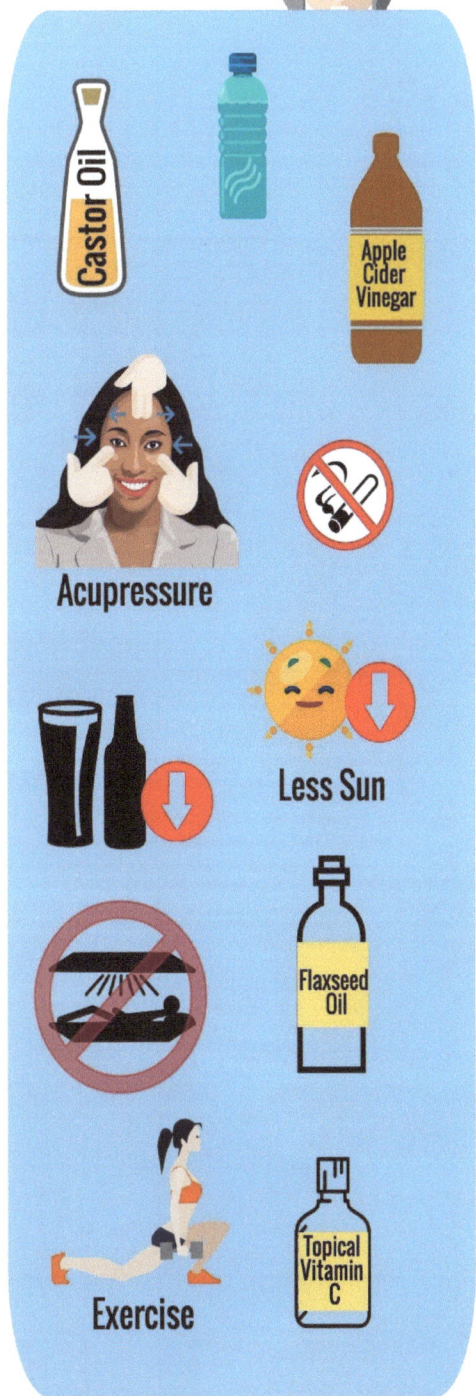

Yeast Infection

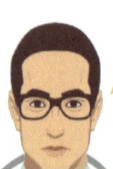
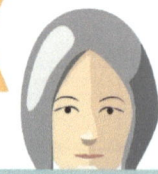

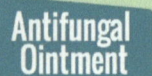
Antifungal Ointment

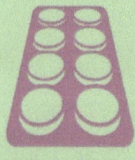
Fluconazole

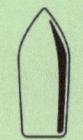
Antifungal Suppository

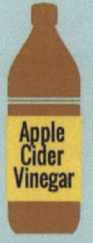
Apple Cider Vinegar

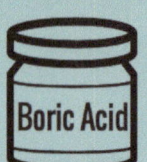
Boric Acid

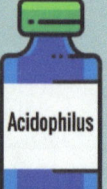
Acidophilus

NO Antibiotics

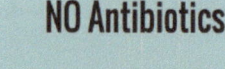

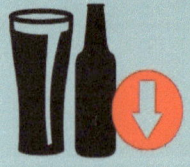

Sugar

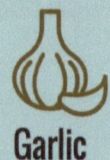
Garlic

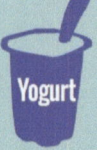
Yogurt

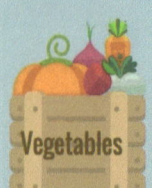
Vegetables

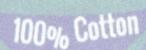
100% Cotton

Sources Used

Here is a partial list of sources used in the making of this book.

Merck Manual

Encyclopedia of Natural Medicine

The Doctor's Book of Home Remedies for Preventing Disease

earthclinic.com

mayoclinic.com

webmd.com

draxe.com

Remember: infographicalremedy.com is the companion site for this book. Do check it out.

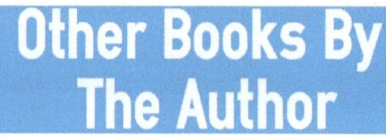

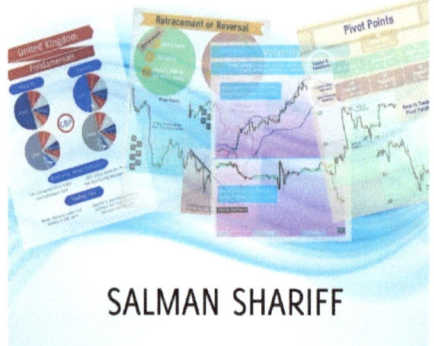

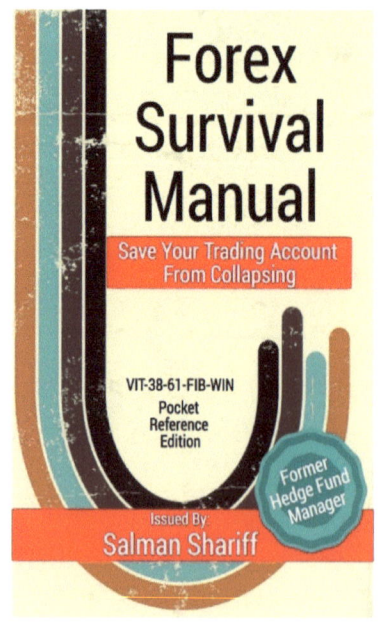

Remedy Journal

Date	Condition	Remedy	Result
Apr 2017	Lack of Health Remedy Knowledge	Infographical Remedy Book	Works Good

Remedy Journal

Date	Condition	Remedy	Result

www.ingramcontent.com/pod-product-compliance
Lightning Source LLC
Chambersburg PA
CBHW041058180526
45172CB00001B/12